Translational Research and Clinical Practice

TRANSLATIONAL RESEARCH AND CLINICAL PRACTICE

Basic Tools for Medical Decision Making and Self-Learning

Stephen C. Aronoff, MD
Waldo E. Nelson Professor and Chairman
Department of Pediatrics
Temple University School of Medicine
Philadelphia, Pennsylvania

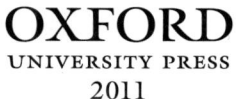

OXFORD
UNIVERSITY PRESS
2011

OXFORD
UNIVERSITY PRESS

Oxford University Press, Inc., publishes works that further
Oxford University's objective of excellence
in research, scholarship, and education.

Oxford   New York
Auckland   Cape Town   Dar es Salaam   Hong Kong   Karachi
Kuala Lumpur   Madrid   Melbourne   Mexico City   Nairobi
New Delhi   Shanghai   Taipei   Toronto

With offices in
Argentina   Austria   Brazil   Chile   Czech Republic   France   Greece
Guatemala   Hungary   Italy   Japan   Poland   Portugal   Singapore
South Korea   Switzerland   Thailand   Turkey   Ukraine   Vietnam

Published by Oxford University Press, Inc.
198 Madison Avenue, New York, New York 10016
www.oup.com

Oxford is a registered trademark of Oxford University Press

Library of Congress Cataloging-in-Publication Data

Aronoff, Stephen C.
Translational research and clinical practice: basic tools for medical decision
making and self-learning / Stephen C. Aronoff.
p. ; cm.
Includes bibliographical references.
ISBN 978-0-19-974644-6
1. Evidence-based medicine.   2. Medicine–Decision making.
3. Clinical trials.   I. Title.
[DNLM: 1. Evidence-Based Practice–methods.   2. Decision Making.
3. Decision Support Techniques.   4. Diagnosis.
5. Translational Research–methods. WB 102.5 A769t 2011]
R723.7.A76 2011
616–dc22
2010018248
ISBN: 978-0-19-974644-6

1 3 5 7 9 8 6 4 2

Printed in the United States of America
on acid-free paper

CONTENTS

PREFACE

When all is said and done, physicians spend most of their time answering four questions raised by their patients: What's wrong with me? Can you treat me? Will I get better? and What caused this?

How physicians answer these questions is as old as the profession itself. From the time of Hippocrates, medical students and residents have been taught by "masters," older, experienced physicians who pass on their skills and knowledge in an apprenticeship-like manner. This method of educating physicians continued to be acceptable until 1910 when Abraham Flexner published his famous report on medical education in the United States. It was this document that set the stage for the educational model that we all know now, the university-based medical school attached to the academic health science center.

While the educational environment for physicians has changed, the method of decision making, in large part, has not. Since the beginning of the profession, many physicians have based their decisions on generalized theories of disease, treatment, and prognosis. These theories advanced by wise, senior practitioners of the art were based on induction and led to the dogmatic school of thought regarding knowledge development. Modern inductive theories have roots in the sciences of molecular and cellular biology, anatomy, physiology, molecular pharmacology, microbiology, immunology, and pathology. Students are still taught to base their medical decisions on inductions derived from these underlying basic science principles. While this is a wonderful way to generate hypotheses for clinical investigation, this method is fraught with problems when applied to clinical issues.

Sextus Empiricus (160–210 AD) was a physician and philosopher with roots in Rome and Athens. Philosophically, he was a skeptic and practiced medicine according to the method that bears his name, empiricism. In ancient times, this school of practice denied theories from induction as a basis for practice. Instead, these practitioners based their care on past experience. Empiricism holds that knowledge arises from experience, emphasizing the role of perception and evidence in this process. The modern iteration of medical empiricism is the reliance on codified, organized experience in the form of translational or clinical research as the basis for medical decision making.

These two schools of thought continue to impact the modern practice of medicine. Today's physicians can draw on two resources to make a clinical decision: *(1)* his or her own unique set of clinical skills, clinical experiences, and knowledge of basic sciences and *(2)* empirical evidence from the medical literature that specifically addresses the issue at hand. The purpose of this book is to focus on the second process. Modern empiricism seeks to draw a narrow inference, complete with an understanding of the associated uncertainty, from translational, clinical research. As opposed to dogmatic thought, modern medical empiricism does not seek to develop broad, dogmatic theories that explain the evolution or etiology of pathological processes; these constructs are left to the basic scientist.

The physician begins the process of medical decision making by obtaining a medical history and performing a physical examination. From this information, the clinician formulates an assessment of the patient's problem. Based on preliminary laboratory information, the physician's knowledge base, and his or her experience, the answer to the question may be readily apparent. When the clinical picture lacks distinguishing features, contains unique exposures or findings, or presents a unique issue of prognosis or therapy, the physician may need to look for specific help from the medical literature. Using a searchable question, the physician must find the appropriate study, determine whether the subjects of the study are similar to the patient at hand, ascertain the outcomes of the study, and finally validate the study. Once this process is complete, a decision can be made regarding the best course of action. For some physicians, the process of question formulation, literature search, and study validation is as much a part of the clinical decision-making process as the physical examination or the medical history.

The skills of information gathering are taught in medical school and honed throughout residency and practice. Although empiricism has roots as ancient as the practice of medicine itself, the modern processes of question formulation, literature search, and study evaluation are relatively new. The formalization of the process began in the 1990s with a series of articles published in *The Journal of the American Medical Association* by David Sackett and his colleagues. The end result is the *User's Guide to the Medical Literature*. This publication can be obtained through *The Journal of the American Medical Association* or found on the Internet at a variety of websites. The techniques for finding, evaluating, and validating studies are detailed there and will be reviewed here in depth. In addition, this book will provide a simple, unified framework for reading and understanding the medical literature.

I am a pediatric infectious disease physician by training. My career has been focused on clinical care, clinical education, and clinical science. I became interested in the use of the medical literature as a patient care tool during my residency at Rainbow Babies and Children's Hospital in Cleveland in the late 1970s. During the time I was a resident, evidence had to be gleaned by hand from hard copies of journals and a catalogue of published articles entitled *Index Medicus*. Finding the guiding evidence was arduous, and we frequently relied on our mentors, Drs. Richard Behrman and William Speck, to guide us to the right answers. Since the delineation of the techniques of evidence-based medicine by Sackett and his colleagues was still 15 years away, we relied on criteria of our own device.

The forum for instruction was intake rounds, a ritual in which the third-year residents presented all of the previous night's admissions to Drs. Behrman and Speck. Following a case presentation, a spirited discussion of management or diagnosis ensued. The presenting resident, who was expected to support any actions taken by evidence from the literature, would present a synopsis of what was found during the night. A typical interaction follows:

Senior resident: I found a paper published 5 years ago in an American journal that says we should do A.

Dr. Speck: There is an article that was published 2 years ago in the British literature that suggests we should do B.

Dr. Behrman: There is an article that is going to be published next month that I reviewed for a journal that says C.

And so it went.

As an educator of medical students and pediatric residents, I have tried to incorporate the use of medical evidence into my daily teaching rounds. By helping the resident or student develop a question for each patient presented at rounds and by giving each student or resident time to find and appraise the evidence that addresses each specific question, I have found that my patients, my residents, and my students have become my teachers. With the development of *(1)* the Internet, *(2)* the National Library of Medicine's Medline database of journals and PubMed Search engine, and *(3)* the codification of the rules of evidence-based medicine, any physician, health care provider or consumer of health care can find the published evidence and determine its impact on patient care. The objective of this book is to provide you, gentle reader, with the tools needed to accomplish this task. I have included many clinical examples so you can see how different types of questions may be answered and the detail that the literature can provide. Because my background is in children's health, many of the examples I have chosen are from that field; I have tried to include other examples to show the broad applicability of these techniques.

This book has its roots in a course I have taught for more than 6 years at Temple University School of Medicine. The first four chapters provide a general framework for developing searchable questions, reading clinical research articles, understanding the design of clinical studies, and developing a useful method for dealing with the uncertainty inherent in all clinical research. The next part of the book deals with the nuts and bolts of answering the most common types of questions that arise in clinical practice: questions of diagnosis, therapy, prognosis, differential diagnosis, clinical presentation, and causality, as well as the use of meta-analyses, clinical guidelines, and clinical prediction rules. The final chapters will present a compact format for presenting clinical evidence and some thoughts for self-learning strategies. The last chapter is for those who may want to teach this course themselves.

As is my prerogative, I would like to thank a number of people who made this book (and my career) possible.

Dr. Richard E. Behrman was Department Chairman at Rainbow Babies and Childrens Hospital in Cleveland. He launched my career in academic medicine by taking the huge risk of appointing me as Chief Resident in Pediatrics for not 1 but 2 years. Many of my colleagues said that he kept me around for a second year to see that I "got it right"; I know it was because I was still at a loss for career goals at the end of the first year. His quiet nature, dedication to his residents and students, and reliance on medical evidence produced an entire generation of pediatric empiricists.

Dr. William T. Speck was program director during my residency, faculty mentor during my fellowship, and chairman during my first academic job. Bill practiced pediatrics by one simple rule: consider it a privilege to care for sick children, not a right. Bill was and is the ultimate skeptic and empiricist. His knowledge of the pediatric literature is encyclopedic and his work ethic served as a model for us all. Over the 10 years he served as Chairman of Pediatrics at Case Western Reserve University, he continued Dr. Behrman's tradition and legacy of training "a lot of really good pediatricians." Many of his trainees are contemporary leaders in their subspecialties; several of us followed the lead of our mentors and became academic department chairs.

Dr. J. Carlton Gartner was a resident and chief resident in pediatrics at Children's Hospital of Pittsburgh and inspired me to enter the field. Carl has a wonderful way with children, students, and residents. Like Drs. Behrman and Speck, he has a remarkable command of the pediatric literature and is a devout empiricist. He taught me the most important lesson I ever learned regarding differential diagnosis: "Common diseases present commonly and common diseases present uncommonly."

I would like to thank my sons, Josh and Matt. Josh has taught me the meaning of courage and perseverance. I will also point out, as a proud father, that Josh did the artwork for the cover of this book. Matt is my hero; his quiet strength and self-reliance are a lesson for all of us. To my dad, a newspaperman who taught me to write "hard and lean," I say thanks for everything.

Finally, I want to thank all of my teachers, current and past; all of the children in Cleveland, Morgantown, and Philadelphia who allowed me to participate in their care and learn from their illnesses; and all of the students and residents in those same places who asked questions that sent all of us scurrying to the literature to find the best evidence. It's been a great ride!

Stephen C. Aronoff, MD
Waldo E. Nelson Professor and Chairman
Department of Pediatrics
Temple University School of Medicine

Translational Research and
Clinical Practice

1

DEVELOPING A CLINICAL QUESTION AND SEARCHING THE MEDICAL LITERATURE

Before you can begin to interpret the medical evidence and apply it to clinical situations, two skills must be mastered: formulating a searchable question and searching the medical literature.

ASKING A QUESTION

Attempting to search the medical literature without a well-defined question is akin to climbing a ladder blindfolded. Once you reach the top, you still have no idea where you are! Searches of the medical literature often begin with one of the four questions patients ask their physicians: *(1)* What's wrong with me (diagnosis)? *(2)* What can you do for me (therapy)? *(3)* Will I get better (prognosis or outcome)? and *(4)* What caused my illness (causality)? To begin, consider the following case scenario:

> A 53-year-old male presents with the complaint of frequency of urination. Over the past several weeks, he has noted difficulty with voiding, voiding more often, and multiple episodes of voiding at night (nocturia). His past medical history and review of systems are not contributory. His father died at the age of 68 of prostatic cancer. Physical examination is normal except for an enlarged, somewhat nodular prostate on rectal examination.

Well-defined, searchable questions consist of several specific elements and begin with a concise description of the patient and the problem. In this case, we can describe the patient as a middle-aged adult male. The problem relates to the patient's complaint of voiding difficulties and can be characterized as frequency of urination and nocturia. We also know that this is associated with prostatic hypertrophy and a family history of prostate cancer. The first order of business is to determine how to distinguish benign prostatic hypertrophy from prostate cancer. We now have all of the elements of a searchable question: *question type* (diagnosis or etiology), *clinical problem* (differentiating prostatic hypertrophy from prostate cancer), and *patient description* (middle-aged male). Putting all of this together, we can ask: "What is the best diagnostic test to differentiate prostatic hypertrophy from prostate cancer in a middle-aged male?"

SEARCHING FOR THE EVIDENCE

Prior to the computer age, searches of the medical literature were done by hand, using a series of books called *Index Medicus*. This series was updated monthly and grouped articles according to MEdical Subject Headings (MESH) terms. The process of thoroughly searching the medical literature took days to weeks. Articles would be identified under the search headings and would be retrieved. Often searches had to be repeated as additional headings were discovered. The bibliographies of identified articles would be searched for more articles. This process required a large amount of time and access to a large medical school library. Literature searches were not something a practitioner away from an academic institution could easily undertake.

Things are much different now. The National Library of Medicine (NLM) maintains a searchable database of the world's medical literature going back to 1966. The database is accessible via the Internet and is free to use. The best search engine for this database is PubMed (http://www.ncbi.nlm.nih.gov/sites/entrez). There are multiple ways to use this search engine.

Main Page

The main page permits the search of several different databases. You can choose which database you want to use by the dropdown menu at the top of the page. The database containing clinical evidence is PubMed. The primary search field is at the top of the page. Words can be searched as groups by enclosing them within quotation marks. Using the question generated in the previous section, we can search, "prostatic hypertrophy," "prostate cancer," and "diagnosis." These three searches have the following outcomes:

- Prostatic hypertrophy: 2558 citations
- Prostate cancer: 42,237 citations
- Diagnosis: over 6 million

Clearly this did not work. However, all is not lost.

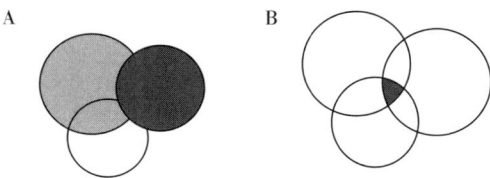

Figure 1-1. Venn diagram of search strategies. (A) Searches of three separate topics. (B) Overlap of the same three topics.

The results using the three search terms are represented by the three circles in Figure 1-1A. This search found every article containing the phrase "prostatic hypertrophy," every article containing the phrase "prostate cancer," and every article containing the word "diagnosis." We are actually interested in the intersection of the three circles as shown in Figure 1-1B. We can generate this search in one of two ways. First, we can combine the three terms in a single search operation separating each phrase with the word AND. AND is called a Boolean operator and requires the search to meet all three conditions. Alternatively, we can click on the hyperlink marked "advanced search." At the top of the page, we find three numbered searches that represent each search already performed. We can click on each search number and the operator AND. The searches are transferred to the query box at the top of the page. Clicking the search key for this query box combines all three searches. The resulting combined search yields 181 citations. Clicking the "advanced search" hyperlink again gives access to the filters and limits page. We select "human" studies, studies in "core journals," studies in "English," and studies among the "middle aged." The result is five studies. The first study is entitled "Free-to-total prostate specific antigen ratio as a single test for detection of significant stage T1c prostate cancer" and was published in the *Journal of Urology* in 1996. This article appears to address our question.

There is another way to perform the same search. Returning to the PubMed home page, click on the hyperlink marked *clinical queries* and go to the *Search by Clinical Study Category* section. Click the radio buttons for *diagnosis* and *narrow search*. When you enter "prostate cancer" in the query box, 180 citations are returned. What we are really interested in are nonsurgical ways to make the diagnosis. We can alter the search using three more Boolean commands. In addition to "prostate cancer," we add the operator NOT. This instructs the search to exclude any articles that include the next term. In fact, we want to add several terms, so we use the following string: NOT (surgery OR molecular OR histol*). This will exclude any articles with the keywords "surgery" or "molecular." The histol* is used to exclude articles with keywords "histology" or "histological." In this way, we can exclude any studies requiring tissue diagnosis. The new search, run through clinical query with *diagnosis* and *narrow search* marked, yielded 69 articles. Among the first seven articles, we find one article that addresses our question: Age adjusted prostate specific antigen and prostate specific antigen velocity cut points in prostate cancer screening. *J Urol* 2007; 177:499. One of the great features of PubMed is that when you click on an article, it brings up additional articles of interest. In this case, five additional papers addressing the diagnostic use of prostate-specific antigen were found.

The clinical queries page contains several other features of interest. Clicking on the *filter table* for the *Search by Clinical Study Category* section shows the difference between narrow and broad search. *Find Systematic Reviews* allows you to search for meta-analyses, a topic to be discussed later. There is also a section on medical genetics.

Using the main search page; the clinical queries page; the Boolean operators AND, NOT, and OR; and the grouping symbols " " and ( ), you should be able to find most of the evidence you will need. On rare occasions, you may need some help with the search strings. On the main page there is a hyperlink marked *MESH database* under the heading *more resources*. Clicking on this page will take you through a simple tutorial for using MESH. These terms are used uniformly by Medline for cataloguing articles. The PubMed search engine usually converts your terms to MESH terms, but not always. When "prostate cancer" is entered into the MESH search engine, the return is prostatic neoplasms. Search strings can be constructed using the MESH search page.

The best way to learn the PubMed search engines is to use them. The features of this page allow you to construct a narrower, more focused search. A Google search of "prostate cancer" yields over 13 million hits, including home pages for many cancer centers. Using Google Scholar for the same search produces 774,000 hits. The Advanced Scholar Search has none of the features of PubMed. Finally, PubMed will provide an abstract of every article and in many cases will provide full-text links to the article itself.

2

THE ANATOMY OF
A CLINICAL STUDY

Like most things in life, clinical studies have a beginning, a middle, and an end. Even though you may find them in one of tens of thousands of journals in a multitude of languages, the anatomy, like that of the human species, is consistent. Each study will have an introduction, methods section, results section, and a discussion or conclusion. Avoid the temptation to just read the conclusion in the abstract; it is not always correct, nor it is phrased in a way that ultimately will be useful. By the end of this chapter, you should be able to read a journal article and find the areas of the article that contain the critical information. The discussion that follows applies to original research articles only, not to review articles, commentaries, or basic science articles that look at results in non-human systems such as bacteria or cell cultures. These articles have their place in providing a context for clinical research but in and of themselves are not applicable directly to medical decision making.

INTRODUCTION

The body of every article starts with an introduction. The introduction provides a one- or two-sentence summary of the topic. The remainder of the introduction includes a brief description of the disease process in question and one or two relevant points regarding the diagnosis, therapy, prognosis, or causality of the disease. The first part of the introduction should provide information about the subject disease and a context for the study. Contained in the last paragraph, often in the last one or two sentences of the last paragraph, is the central hypothesis of the study. This part of the introduction should contain a succinct statement of the specific aims of the study. Consider the last sentence in this example:

> The Avoiding Cardiovascular Events through Combination Therapy in Patients Living with Systolic Hypertension (ACCOMPLISH) trial was designed to test the hypothesis that treatment with an ACE inhibitor combined with amlodipine would result in better cardiovascular outcomes than treatment with the same ACE inhibitor combined with a thiazide diuretic. (*N Engl J Med* 2008; 359:2417)

Besides a really catchy but somewhat corny acronym, you know that *(1)* this is a study that addresses a therapeutic issue, *(2)* there will be a comparison between two groups of patients, one group receiving ACE inhibitor plus amlodipine and one group receiving ACE inhibitor plus thiazide diuretic, and *(3)* the outcome of the trial will be some kind of cardiovascular event or events. You also know that this article was published in the *New England Journal of Medicine* in 2008, and it can be found in volume 359 beginning on page 2417. If you cannot find a statement similar to this or if it is not sufficiently detailed to draw these kinds of conclusions, consider finding another article. Each piece of significant medical evidence should have a well-defined objective.

METHODS

The methods sections of clinical reports contain several subsections. As you read through this part of the paper, you want to identify four things: *(1)* patient population or subjects; *(2)* investigational therapies, tests, or risk factors; *(3)* comparative therapy, gold standard test, or baseline conditions; and *(4)* primary outcome of the study. The mnemonic PICO is often used to describe this part of the study. Let's look at these components in detail.

Patient Population or Subjects

If there is no description of the patient population, there is not much point in continuing to read the study. We are only interested in studies that look at human subjects, not experimental systems like cell lines or animal studies. The description of those patients included in the study should be complete and detailed. The characteristics of the patient population can be thought of in terms of a general description, inclusion criteria, exclusion criteria, and method of selection.

The *general description* of the subject population is largely demographic. Ages (pediatric versus adult), location, and the typical clinical presentation should be easy to find. For example, in the hypertension study cited in the previous section, the subjects were drawn from "...five countries (U.S., Sweden, Norway, Denmark, and Finland), representing

548 centers." In all cases, there should be a statement that informed consent was obtained from each subject or was deemed unnecessary and that the protocol was reviewed by an institutional review board for the protection of human subjects.

The *inclusion criteria* should be detailed so that you can determine exactly which patient conditions were included in the study. In many cases this may limit the applicability of the results of the study. In the hypertension example, the following statement was made:

> All enrolled patients had hypertension and were at high risk for cardiovascular events; patients were included who had a history of coronary events, myocardial infarction, revascularization, or stroke; impaired renal function; peripheral artery disease; left ventricular hypertrophy; or diabetes mellitus.

Reading further, you find that hypertension was defined as blood pressure exceeding 140/90. The inclusion criteria should provide a definition of the primary disease process (in this case a blood pressure greater than 140/90) and any other factors that must be present to be included in the study.

Now, you may not know what all of these conditions are, but you do know that this was not a study of relatively healthy people with newly diagnosed hypertension. So if your patient does not have any of these risk factors, stop reading. This study is not applicable. Similarly, the results of this study do not apply to women who become hypertensive during pregnancy (preeclampsia) or to children with hypertension.

The *exclusion criteria*, when present, should be as detailed as the inclusion criteria. For example, in a study designed to assess the risk of recurrent seizures after a seizure without fever in children without underlying disease or injury, those subjects with "typical absence seizures, myoclonic seizures, and infantile spasms as well as those who presented with their first generalized tonic-clonic seizure but were found to have had prior absence, myoclonic, or partial seizures" were excluded (*Pediatrics* 1996; 98:216). These authors went to great lengths to exclude a variety of seizure types. The goal of the study was to assess those risk factors for future seizures in otherwise normal children who are seen by physicians for simple, uncomplicated seizures. While this provides very good data for the population studied, if your patient had an absence seizure, these data are not applicable.

The *method of selection* of subjects as well as the venue where the patients are first seen can influence the outcome of a study. In general, the more random the selection process, the better. In some studies, consecutive patients who present for care over a given period of time are used. In other studies, hospital records are searched for patients with a specific diagnosis. In the latter case, you lose all of the patients who were not admitted to hospital. This is important since it excludes patients who were managed as outpatients or those who died before admission. The venue of care is also important. The severity of disease and, as a result, potential differences in outcome occur among patients seen in a private doctor's office compared with those who may be seen in the emergency department of a large urban hospital.

Investigational and Comparative Therapy, Test or Risk Factors

As we will see in the next chapter, most clinical studies involve a comparison between two groups of subjects. In the case of therapy, it may be a group that received a new therapy compared to a group that received standard therapy or no therapy at all (placebo). In the case of a new diagnostic test, it may be a comparison of the performance of a new test with that of an old one or one that is considered a "gold standard" (a test that defines a given disease state). In other studies, patients will be assigned to different groups based on the presence or absence of given factors or, in the parlance of epidemiology, exposures. Most modern clinical studies compare outcomes among multiple groups. We will discuss this in detail later.

Outcome

Each study should have a single event or condition designated as the *primary outcome*. The design of modern clinical studies is based around a single primary outcome. Often, this outcome represents a dichotomous parameter: the number of patients who died or survived; the number of patients who developed a significant complication; the number of patients requiring hospitalization. These types of outcomes (yes or no) are easy to understand, have clinical relevance, and are easy to remember. In other cases, the primary outcome may be a continuous parameter such as height, weight, blood pressure, total white blood cell count, and so on. A valid clinical study will identify a single metric as its primary outcome.

Many studies, particularly therapeutic trials, also have secondary outcomes. For example, in an HIV clinical drug trial, the primary outcome may be the death rate, while secondary outcomes may include changes in viral load, CD_4 count, and rates of opportunistic infections. In another example, the primary outcome may be the death rate for the total population enrolled in the study, and secondary outcomes may be the rate in subpopulations such as women, children, or individuals with low CD_4 counts. In all of these instances, the secondary outcomes embellish the story; the real tale lies with the primary outcome.

Differences in outcomes can be determined from a 2×2 table (Fig. 2-1). As an example, assume that the outcome is a negative event, such as death, and that the treatment group had a lower death rate than the placebo group. The death rate for the treatment group ($n = a + b$) is $R_t = a/(a + b)$; the death rate for the control group ($n = c + d$) is $R_c = c/(c + d)$. Assume R_c is $> R_t$. How can we compare these two rates in order to make a judgment regarding clinical efficacy?

	Outcome Event: Present	Outcome Event: Absent
Treatment Group	a	b
Control Group	c	d

Figure 2-1. 2 x 2 Box used to determine outcome rates from clinical trials. $R_t = a/(a + b)$; $R_c = c/(c + d)$.

The *rate ratio (RR) or likelihood ratio (LR) or Bayesian factor* is defined by the ratio of the outcome rate in the control group to that of the treatment group: R_c/R_t. In this case, the ratio would be greater than 1, suggesting that the relative "risk" of dying is higher in the control group. The ratio could also be inverted to show that the "risk" of dying would be lower in the treatment group. Rate ratios express the outcome as the relative weight of data supporting one hypothesis to another mutually exclusive hypothesis, are easy to understand, and permit the direct determination of clinical significance. To me, this is the best way to express outcome results, and it is used extensively throughout the remainder of this book.

Absolute risk reduction (ARR) is the difference in outcome rates between the two groups: $R_c - R_t$. Because this expression permits calculations of number needed to treat (1/ARR), it is used extensively in clinical trials. *Relative risk reduction* is defined as the difference in outcome rates between the two groups as a proportion of the outcome rate in the control group: ARR/R_c. Relative risk reduction is often used to define vaccine efficacy. For example, if a vaccine is described as 95% effective, the difference in rates of infection between the vaccines and the controls is 95% of the rate in the control group.

Odds ratios (ORs) or relative odds are defined as the odds of dying for the control group divided by the odds of dying for the treatment group. The odds of dying for the treatment group (O_t) is defined as a/b (Fig. 2-1); for the control group, $O_c = c/d$. The odds ratio = O_c/O_t. Although the odds ratio is more versatile mathematically, it is difficult to understand conceptually. If the RR is 1.5, we know that the death rate in the placebo group was 50% higher than the rate in the treatment group. That is not true for an odds ratio of 1.5. Interpretation of odds ratios is shown in Figure 2-2.

Odds Ratio Range	Favors H_0 over H_1
>100	Decisive
32–100	Very strong
10–32	Strong
3.2–10	Substantial
1.3.2	"not worth more than a mention"
.31–1	"not worth more than a mention"
.1–.31	Substantial
.03–.1	Strong
.01	Very strong
<.01	Decisive

Figure 2-2.   Clinical interpretation of odds ratios.(Reprinted with permission from Jeffreys, H. *Theory of probability.* Oxford University Press, Oxford, 1961.)

Statistical Analysis

For the most part, you can ignore this section. It is typically incomprehensible to most readers. In the case of a therapeutic or a randomized trial, you want to look at a power calculation to make sure the study is sized appropriately; you also want to make sure that whatever assumptions went into that calculation are borne out by the results. We will provide much more on this topic later.

RESULTS

The results sections of most clinical studies are straightforward, centered on tables and graphs, and follow a clear format. The initial part of the discussion should focus on the number, demographics, and the baseline characteristics of the subjects. In the case of a randomized trial, the two groups should be compared with regard to demographics and baseline characteristics to prove that the randomization scheme worked.

The next part of the study should show the results for the primary outcome. In any event, that is the part of the study you should look for next, since it is pivotal. The following chapters will discuss this in great detail, since this is the critical bottom line of any study. The results section should end with secondary outcomes and any post hoc analyses of subgroups.

DISCUSSION

All clinical studies end with a discussion or conclusions section. With the tools you will learn here, this section should be largely irrelevant. From the methods and results sections you should be able to draw your own conclusions. For your purpose, the discussion section should be a post script, that is, the author's *opinion* as to how the trial should be interpreted and how it fits into the grand scheme of things. The author should leave you with a sense as to the existing gaps in current knowledge regarding the topic, what additional studies may be needed, and how the present study answers previous questions.

3

DESIGNS OF CLINICAL STUDIES

The central feature of any study and a major point of the Methods section of any paper is a description of the study design. Before we start, a word about bias. In this context, bias represents the potential introduction of error into a study. Bias may be introduced systematically or randomly. Systematic bias affects the outcome of the study. For example, if the investigator of a study is allowed to choose who gets the new therapy and who gets the old, the possibility exists that she may subconsciously administer the new therapy only to those patients she thinks will be most responsive. This is an example of selection bias. Conversely, if the investigator is blinded as to the drug assignment, those patients not given the new therapy are given a placebo (a pill that looks like the experimental drug), and the assignment of patients to groups is determined randomly, then, at worst, she will introduce random bias. The reason modern clinical studies are randomized and blinded is that any unknown factor that may affect the outcome (covariate) should be equally distributed between the two groups; in this way, covariate effects are cancelled or minimized.

Each study can be categorized by its timing and its grouping. The *timing* of a study refers to whether the subjects and data were gathered *prospectively* (forward in time) or *retrospectively* (backward in time) with regard to the outcome. Prospective studies define the population of subjects (sometimes called a cohort) and the investigational protocol prior to the initiation of data gathering. These studies have the advantage of ensuring that a random sample of patients will be enrolled (selection bias), that complete data will be collected in real time (recall bias), and that patients have been observed or treated prior to the primary outcome event (cause-effect bias). Retrospective studies define the subject population and the investigational protocol after the outcome has occurred. Most of these studies will use hospital records or preexisting databases as the data source. Since the patients have already come and gone, records may be incomplete or patients may have to remember facts that occurred in the distant past (recall bias); subjects may be missed by the search of the records, or only those patients who were admitted to hospital may be included in the study (selection bias); or events may be transposed since the outcome of interest has already occurred (cause-effect bias).

Clinical studies also may be grouped as noncomparative or comparative. Noncomparative studies include only one group of patients, while comparative studies include two or more groups. *Noncomparative studies* include case reports and case series. Case studies often report new or unusual associations, detailed evaluations of unusual diseases (often metabolic or immunological in nature), new surgical procedures, unusual complications of drug therapy, and novel clinical presentations. As one of my mentors used to say, a case study says "we saw this" or "we did this."

Retrospective case series have a number of clinical applications. One of the most important case series was a report in the late 1970s of a clustering of cases of Kaposi's sarcoma, a rare cutaneous tumor, among gay men in California. This was the first clinical report of acquired immune deficiency syndrome (AIDS). A collection of patients with a rare or unusual disease is also useful for understanding the spectrum of associated symptoms as well as the natural history of the disease. For example, in 1980 the Centers for Disease Control and Prevention (CDC) reported a series of 261 children who met the clinical diagnostic criteria for Kawasaki disease (*Pediatrics* 1980; 65:21). From this study we learned that *(1)* the disease is unusual in children over 8 years of age; *(2)* the disease occurs mostly in previously healthy children; *(3)* all of the children present with fever, 98% with rashes, 96% with conjunctival injection, and 81% with lymphadenopathy; and *(4)* arthralgias occur in 55% and diarrhea in 48%. There are much more data regarding the prevalence of different symptoms and laboratory values in this population. From a natural history point of view, these largely untreated children had a 15% incidence of cardiac complications, 9% incidence of pulmonary infiltrates, 26% incidence of cerebrospinal fluid pleocytosis (white blood cells in the cerebrospinal fluid), and rare episodes of gallbladder disease, hair loss, and paralytic ileus.

Large case series are useful for developing differential diagnoses. For example, a 13-year-old boy was admitted to our hospital for the evaluation of long-standing respiratory disease. His sister had the same thing. Computed tomography of the chest demonstrated bronchiectasis. The most common cause of childhood bronchiectasis is cystic fibrosis; however, both his and his sister's DNA tests for cystic fibrosis were negative. A case series of 136 British children with bronchiectasis not caused by cystic fibrosis was reported in 2005 (*Eur Respir J* 2005; 26:8). Immune problems accounted for 34%, recurrent aspiration pneumonia for 26%, primary ciliary dykinesia for 22%, and structural abnormalities for 3%, and 26% of the subjects went undiagnosed. This paper pointed us in the right direction, and a primary immunodeficiency was found in both this boy and his sister.

Case series and case reports are *not* useful for assessing outcomes of therapy, utility of diagnostic tests, or for determining causality. These types of studies constitute anecdotal evidence. Since there is no comparative group to control for covariates or coincidental occurrences, nondescriptive conclusions from these types of studies are highly subject to the fallacy of *post hoc ergo propter hoc*, literally "after this, therefore, because of this." For example, a 15-month-old boy is diagnosed with autism 1 month after he receives a live, attenuated mumps, measles, and rubella vaccine. Some would conclude that the vaccine caused the disorder, but consider this. More than 80% of all American children between 12 and 15 months of age receive this vaccine. The incidence of autism is approximately 1/2000 children, and most of these children manifest symptoms of the disorder between 1 and 2 years of age. Given the overlap of ages of these two events and the large number of children who receive the vaccine and have autism, it is not unexpected that some of these affected children will coincidentally be diagnosed with autism in proximity to receipt of the vaccine. This is called *survivor bias*, and it is discussed in detail in Chapter 4. Clearly a different kind of study is required to determine causality.

There are a variety of *comparative study designs*, all with their own advantages, disadvantages, and uses. The study types will be presented in order of increasing reliability and strength.

A *case-control* study, like most case series, is performed backward in time. Cases are identified as the result of an event or disease. Controls, individuals who do not have the disease or have not suffered the event of interest, are matched to the cases based on age, sex, and other demographics. Using preexisting records from a database, information is gathered and risk factors are identified that may have an increased frequency of occurrence among the case subjects when compared to the controls. Outcomes can only be expressed as a rate ratio or likelihood ratio (Chapter 2). These types of studies are useful in situations where an event has already occurred (such as an outbreak of an infectious disease) and the risk factors for the event can only be identified in retrospect. Case-control studies are also used when the event of interest occurs rarely. The studies linking cigarette smoking and lung cancer were case-control studies. These types of studies have several important limitations. *Recall bias* is the greatest problem. Since these studies are performed backward in time, recalling exposure to selected factors months or years prior may be difficult. *Selection bias* is also a problem since it is difficult to find control individuals who match the case subjects in all aspects. Finally, the direction of the study, effect to cause, is a major limitation to the strength of the inference that can be drawn from these types of studies.

Retrospective cohort studies utilize large, preexisting databases often generated by federal agencies, large health systems, or hospitals. In many cases, the databases are not set up specifically to answer a research question. For example, several recent studies have identified patients and data using hospital billing databases. Questions are asked by extracting data and setting up comparisons among subgroups within the database. Since this is a retrospective design, these studies have the same limitations as case-control studies. Data from these kinds of studies are sometimes used to identify issues that need to be evaluated more rigorously.

Unlike the other studies discussed to this point, *cohort or observational studies* are performed forward in time. The design of these studies is straightforward. A group of patients (cohort) is defined and gathered at the onset of the study. Informational data are collected forward in time until a previously defined event occurs or sufficient time has elapsed to preclude occurrence of the endpoint event. Data are then analyzed based on occurrence/nonoccurrence of the primary outcome event. This type of study is used to answer questions of diagnosis, prognosis, and etiology, and to develop clinical prediction rules. Unlike the designs previously described, cohort studies may take long periods of time to complete. If the event of interest is rare, prohibitively large numbers of patients may need to be followed in order to obtain clinically significant results. As such, these studies may be expensive to perform.

Clinical trials are typically used to address issues of therapeutic efficacy or treatment and are performed forward in time. Patients are randomly assigned to the experimental agent or to standard therapy or a placebo. Both the investigator and the subject are blinded to the nature of the treatment that each individual receives ("double blinded"). A primary outcome parameter is defined for each study. Most of these studies are of parallel design: patients are randomized at the start to the study arm (experimental therapy) or the control arm (placebo or standard therapy). The subjects are followed longitudinally until the outcome or a time endpoint is reached. A cross-over study design requires that each subject receive both the control and the experimental agents during separate time intervals. These intervals are separated by a "washout" period. The parallel design requires more patients and a larger sample size. The cross-over design is limited by the length of the washout period and the bias of prior effect (extension of a therapeutic effect from the initial treatment period into the second placebo or treatment period). For example, patients who are randomized to receive the experimental agent during the first period may have better outcomes at the end of the placebo period due to carryover of treatment response, lessening the effect size and reducing the likelihood of finding significant differences between the experimental agent and the placebo. Experimental studies are limited by cost and sample size. In particular, if the effect size (difference in outcome between the experimental group and the control group) is small or the outcome in the placebo group is uncommon, the sample size will be large. Dropouts and noncompliance with experimental protocols further affect the interpretation of randomized clinical trials.

Meta-analyses, or systematic reviews, are literally studies of studies. Meta-analyses are often used to expand the power of small clinical trials. Using an a priori protocol and well-defined inclusion criteria, meta-analyses permit the pooling of data from multiple studies. The criteria for the performance of these studies are strict and will be discussed in detail later.

4

LIES, MORE LIES, AND
STATISTICS (WITH
APOLOGIES TO MARK
TWAIN)

Two logical processes connect experimental data and the greater rule or hypothesis that governs the behavior of the facts. Reasoning from the rule to the specific facts is called deduction and is a characteristic of legal arguments. Induction is the process through which one reasons from the specific facts to the general hypothesis or rule. Inductive reasoning is the process used to draw conclusions from clinical research and apply data in medical decision making.

The science of statistics is intimately connected to medical decision making. Unfortunately, the way statistics are used in modern medical research answers a question that is largely irrelevant to clinical practice. Consider a traditional clinical trial where one group of patients receives treatment and the other group receives a placebo. An appropriate clinical outcome is identified and measured in both groups. Assuming a dichotomous outcome (e.g., cures vs. failures), outcome rates (cured/total patients in group) can be calculated for the treatment group (O_t) and the placebo group (O_p). As we will discuss later in this chapter, the preferred summary measurement for this type of study is the ratio of cure rates between the two treatment groups called the *rate ratio* or *likelihood ratio*, O_t/O_p. A traditional statistical argument would be: if there is no difference between the two rates, then $O_t = O_p$ and $O_t/O_p = 1$. If, $O_t > O_p$, then we can conclude that the data support the hypothesis that treatment is better than the placebo. Conversely, if $O_t < O_p$, then we can conclude that the data do not support the hypothesis that the treatment is superior. If the outcome were expressed as a difference in rates, $O_t - O_p$, and there is no difference

21

between the two rates, then $O_t = O_p$ and $O_t - O_p = 0$. The remaining arguments would be identical.

Regardless of how the outcome is expressed, the actual rates for the two groups can be easily calculated from the experimental data. The conclusion from the study would be very easy to find except for one fact: we cannot test the entire population of patients who qualify for a study like this. The use of a sample drawn from the total population of potential subjects introduces uncertainty into the determination of each rate. How much uncertainty is a function of the number of patients included in the study (sample size) and is defined by the *standard deviation*. The derivation and calculation of this value are not important to this discussion. It *is* important to realize that in most of the clinical studies that you read, the outcome of the study will be summarized by a *measure of central tendency* (in our example, this would be the rate ratio or absolute difference calculated from the experimental data) and the *standard deviation* of that measure. In the case of our example and in all of the cases you will encounter in the medical literature, both of these measures are required to determine whether a difference actually exists between the two groups. The way statistics are used in modern research answers the question: "How certain can I be that a difference exists?" Statistics do not answer the questions: "How large is that difference?" and "How certain can I be of that difference?" To understand the limitations of statistics, we need to consider the two conventional theories of statistical thought: Fisher's *p* value and the Neyman–Pearson theory.

FISHER'S *p* VALUE

In almost every study you read, a summary statistic is used to express the degree of certainty that two groups are different. The best known of these is the *p value*. The *p* value was described in 1925 by R. A. Fisher when he suggested the use of a boundary between statistical significance and insignificance. The *p* value, then, was defined as the probability that the observed data occurred by chance. He arbitrarily chose a value of 5% (.05), a choice that lives on today. Thus, the *p* value is only a test of significance and a measurement of error, not a test that chooses one hypothesis over the other. The calculation of the *p* value is directly dependent on sample size. As the sample size increases for a given *p* value, $p = .04$ for example, the differences between study groups become smaller. A simple example illustrates this point. Assume we ask patients to choose between two options, A and B, and let's set $p = .04$. Table 4-1 illustrates the impact of sample size, called the *Lindley paradox*, on the differences between the two groups. At its extreme, a "significant difference" is found when the two groups differ by only .14%!

The *p* value also suffers from "survivor bias." Assume, for example, that 100 people suffer from a disease that has a 5% survival rate after 10 years. You follow the cohort forward in time and, sure enough, only 5 of

Table 4-1. Four Theoretical Studies, All with the Same Two-Sided p Value for the Null Hypothesis of Equal Preference in the Population

Total No. of Patients Receiving A and B	Nos. Preferring A:B	Percent Preferring A	Two-Tailed p Value
20	15:5	75	.04
200	115:86	57.5	.04
2000	1046:954	52.3	.04
2,000,000	1,001,445:998,555	50.07	.04

Source. Reprinted with permission from Spiegelhalter DJ, Abrams KR, Myles JP. *Bayesian approaches to clinical trials and health-care evaluation.* Hoboken, NJ: Wiley, 2004.

the original 100 are alive. Any factor that may be arbitrarily associated with this group (e.g., they all like apples) may prove to be a statistically significant factor for survival ($p = .05!$).

NEYMAN–PEARSON THEORY

In 1950, Neyman developed a statistical method for using data to choose between two mutually exclusive courses of action. Each course of action was defined explicitly by a hypothesis; one of the hypotheses was chosen as the test hypothesis (H_o) and the other as the alternate hypothesis (H_A). Historically, the test hypothesis is the null hypothesis and for our example using the rate ratio would be defined as H_o: $O_t/O_p = 1$ or the equivalent statement $O_t = O_p$. Extending the example, H_A: $O_t \neq O_p$. Following the example of the p value, this method tests the statistical significance of both hypotheses. The test for H_o is called the α *value* and it behaves in a fashion identical to the p value (Fig. 4-1). Also like the p value, for most studies $\alpha = .05$ is set as the level of significance, is determined directly from the experimental evidence, and represents the probability of falsely rejecting H_o. A second statistic, β, defines the probability of falsely rejecting H_A. The mathematical description of this statistic is more complicated, but it is a function of the sample size and of the effect size (the expected difference between O_t and O_p). In most studies that you read, a value for $1 - \beta$, called *power*, is given; this value is usually set at .80 to .90 and is estimated a priori in order to determine the size of the sample needed for the investigation. At the end of the study, based on the calculated values for α and β, a decision can be made as to which course of action the data supports.

THE PROBLEM WITH p, α, AND β VALUES

Although you will see the results from studies expressed in terms of p, α, and β, it is not always clear what conclusion can be drawn. The source of this dilemma is that the p value and the Neyman–Pearson theory summarize experimental data as a probability of an error function, not the

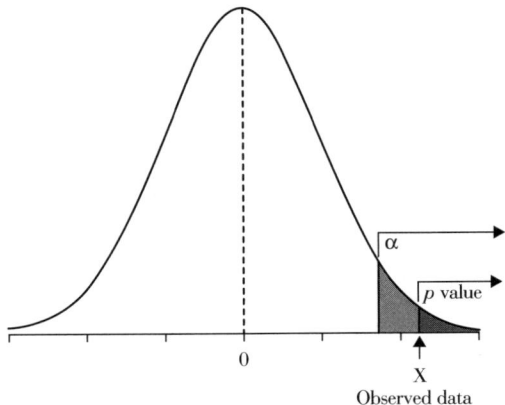

Figure 4-1. Relationship of α and *p* values in a normalized, Gaussian distribution. (Reprinted with permission from Goodman, SN. Toward evidence-based medical statistics. 1: The *p* value fallacy. *Ann Intern Med* 1999; 130:995–1004.)

probability of a given outcome. If only a *p* value (equivalent to α in the hypothesis testing theory) is given, no conclusion can be drawn if *p* > .05, since the test of significance has not been met. If *p* < .05, then you can conclude that the data do not support the null hypothesis or that some unusual event has occurred; without a power calculation or other expression of β, there is no way of determining what, if any, support exists for H_A. If the β condition is met, then conclusions can be drawn regarding the potential risk of error of selecting one hypothesis over the other. Again, no measure of the magnitude or strength of the evidence (clinical significance) is given. In our example, if the value and standard deviation of O_t/O_p is such that *p* < .05 with a sample and effect size such that $1 - β = .80$, we can conclude with some certainty that $O_t \neq O_p$. How big this difference and its direction remain unknown.

THE LIKELIHOOD PRINCIPLE

No two ways about it: *p* values, α, and β are confusing. There must be a simpler way to decide if a real, clinically significant difference exists between two sample populations. Let's look first at how the outcome of the study should be expressed.

As noted in Chapter 2, there are several ways that the outcome rates between two different study groups may be expressed: the difference between the two rates (*absolute rate reduction* or *rate difference*), the ratio of the odds of the two rates (*odds ratio*), the difference between the two rates divided by the rate in the control group (*relative risk reduction*), and the ratio of the two rates (*likelihood ratio* or *rate ratio*). What, then, is the best method for expressing the outcome of a study?

The law of likelihood is the result of a complex mathematical derivation. If you want to "look under the hood," consider reading Richard Royall's treatise entitled "Statistical Evidence: A Likelihood Paradigm" (Chapman and Hall/CRC, New York, 1997). The law of likelihood states that the outcome of any comparative study can be summarized by the ratio of outcomes where each outcome rate represents a mutually exclusive hypothesis. Consider a simple example. Assume that R_p represents the death rate in a group of patients who received a placebo, while R_T represents the death rate of a comparable group of patients who received an active drug. The outcome of this study can be summarized by the ratio R_p/R_T. Moreover, R_p is a proxy for the hypothesis that the placebo is superior and R_T is a proxy for the hypothesis that drug therapy is superior, two mutually exclusive hypotheses. As a result, the likelihood ratio, R_p/R_T, provides a direct, summary measure of how strongly the data support one hypothesis over the other.

CONFIDENCE INTERVALS

Expressing the outcome of a clinical study as a likelihood ratio is only the beginning. The outcome of any study is summarized not only by the measure of central tendency but by the standard deviation around that value. The measure of central tendency and its standard deviation together summarize the data and its inherent uncertainty. If we make one assumption, that these data behave in a normal fashion, then we can generate a likelihood probability function using these two values. This probability function is familiar and is known as a *normal* or *Gaussian distribution*.

Let's look at an example. A recent study looked at the efficacy of a vaccine made from cytomegalovirus envelope glycoprotein b (*N Engl J Med* 2009; 360:1191). In this study 234 susceptible women received the vaccine and 230 susceptible women received a placebo. The subjects were followed for 42 months and the primary endpoint was cytomegalovirus infection; there were 18/234 infections among vaccine recipients (O_t) and 31/230 infections in those who received the placebo (O_p). If we look at the infection rates and express them as a likelihood ratio (O_p/O_t), we can calculate a central value of 1.8 and a standard deviation of .31. The probability function for this study is shown in Figure 4-2.

Is the vaccine superior to the placebo? In the paper, the authors state that the vaccine recipients are less likely to become infected than those who received the placebo ($p = .02$). Power ($1 - \beta$) was calculated at .8. Now what can you conclude? You can say with 98% certainty that the hypothesis that the effect of the vaccine is equal to that of the placebo is incorrect and with 80% certainty that the hypothesis that the vaccine is superior to the placebo is true. This tells us nothing about the magnitude of the effect (clinical significance).

In Figure 4-2, the arrow shows the central value for the curve, 1.8. The line at 1 indicates the point of indifference, where the vaccine and

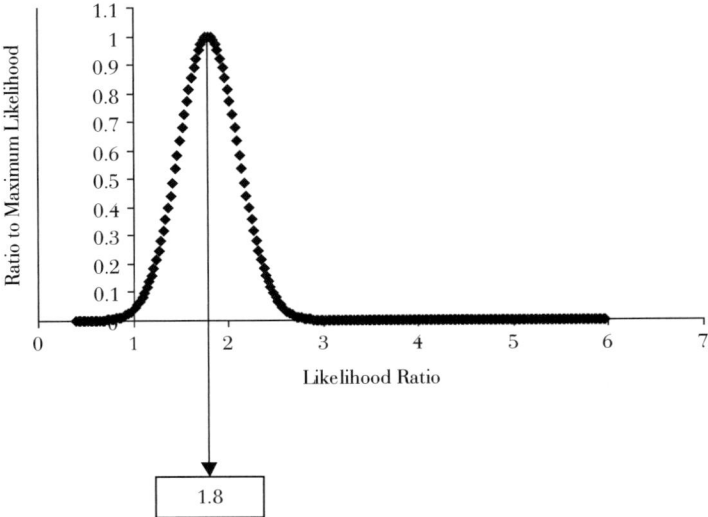

Figure 4-2. Probability function for the cytomegalovirus infection rate ratio of unvaccinated to vaccinated susceptible women. Value for central tendency = 1.8.

placebo are equally effective; the area to the right of 1 favors the vaccine over the placebo, while the area to the left favors the placebo over the vaccine. Simple inspection of Figure 4-2 suggests that most of the curve lies to the right of 1, consistent with the conclusion we drew from the statistics.

The beauty of the normal distribution is that the curve follows precise mathematical rules and permits assumptions about the distribution of the data. We know that the area to the right of the central value encompasses 50% of the curve. We can conclude that 50% of the data supports a rate ratio of 1.8 or greater. We can restate that to say that 50% of the data supports an infection rate that is 80% (1.8 − 1) or greater for placebo recipients than for vaccine recipients. Unfortunately, that also means that 50% of the data supports an infection rate of 80% or less among the placebo recipients as compared to the vaccinees. We have the right elements in the statement, but things are too ambiguous as they stand.

Another property of the normal curve is that the "probability density" at any point can be calculated. Consider Figure 4-3. At a point 1.65 standard deviations below the central point, 95% of the data will lie to the right. In this case, 1.8 − (1.65 × .31) is 1.28. Using this information, we can conclude that 95% of the data supports a 28% (1.28 − 1) or greater infection rate among placebo recipients as compared to vaccinees. That's a convincing statement! Looking at the top end, 1.8 + (1.65 × .31) tells us that 95% of the data supports an infection rate among the placebo recipients no more than 2.3 times that of the vaccinees. Together, these two

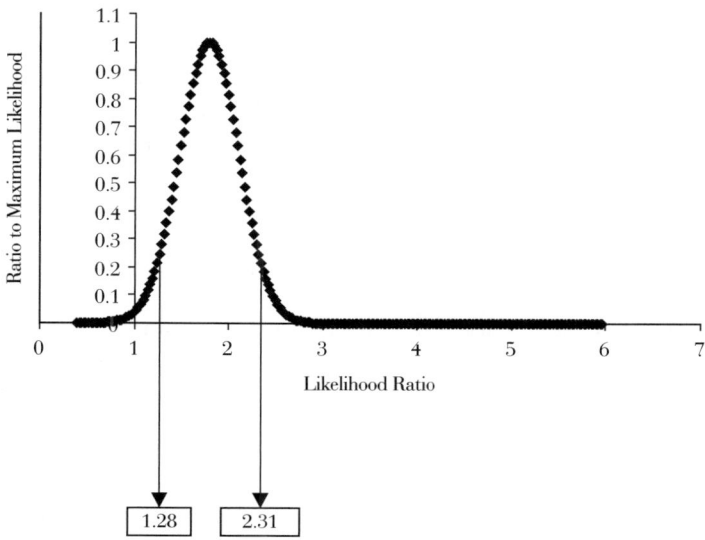

Figure 4-3. Probability function for the cytomegalovirus infection rate ratio of unvaccinated to vaccinated susceptible women. Lower 95% boundary = 1.28; upper 95% boundary = 2.31.

values, 1.28 and 2.31, comprise a *confidence interval.* From the reasoning presented earlier, we know that 5% of the data lies to the *left* of 1.28 (the lower limit of the confidence interval) and 5% of the data lies to the *right* of 2.31 (the upper limit of the confidence interval); since 90% of the data lies between these two values, we would refer to this as the *90% confidence interval.*

CLINICAL SIGNIFICANCE REQUIRES A NEW "POINT OF REFERENCE"

If we can calculate 90% confidence intervals, it should be apparent that we can calculate confidence intervals of any size as long as we know the central value and the standard deviation. What size of confidence interval is appropriate for determining clinical effectiveness? To answer this question, let's begin with how intervals are commonly reported.

In most studies that you read in medical journals, you will find either the central value + the standard deviation or the central value and the lower and upper values for a 95% confidence interval. These limits are 1.96 (conveniently rounded to 2) standard deviations below and above the central value, respectively. Why is a 95% confidence interval used? Remember Sir Roland Fisher of *p* value fame? He gave us the concept of the 5% error as the threshold for statistical significance. In cases where the results of the study are expressed as a rate ratio or an odds ratio, if the 95% confidence interval does not include 1 then there is a statistically significant difference between the two groups. In the case of rate differences, if 0 is not included in the 95% confidence interval, we can draw the same conclusion. So while 95% is a great number for statistical significance, is it an appropriate number for clinical significance?

Let's add another piece to this puzzle. When we look at statistical significance, we are interested in whether the point of indifference (1 or 0) is included in the interval. When we think about clinical significance, we want the difference between the two groups to be more than trivial. In the case of a therapeutic study, we may require a minimum difference of 15% to 25% between therapies or between treatment and placebo to be convincing. In the case of a study looking at adverse outcomes, we may choose to lower that threshold to 4%. In any event, our point of reference for clinical significance is markedly different from the point of reference (0 or 1) for statistical significance.

Therefore, to determine clinical significance, we need to define the point of reference. Since we look at this reference point as a threshold boundary (we want the therapeutic effectiveness to exceed 15% or the risk of harm to be less than 4%, for example) only one boundary of the interval holds our interest.

One of the quirks of traditional statistics is the use of the 95% confidence interval. While this interval includes 95% of the data, 2.5% of the data lies above the upper confidence limit and 2.5% of the data lies below the lower confidence interval. From a clinical significance point of view, we are interested in only one boundary of the interval. We can set this interval at whatever level we choose, but if we choose to set the boundary so that 95% of the data is included, 5%, not 2.5% of the data needs to lie outside of the single boundary. As a result, 90% intervals are much more useful to the clinician than 95% intervals.

THE PREPONDERANCE OF EVIDENCE

Our legal colleagues use the term "preponderance of evidence" as a standard to decide guilt in civil law suits. If you ask a lawyer (I have, my wife), she will define this as "most of the evidence" or "much more than 50% of the evidence." Because of the nature of the normal distribution, we can be as precise as we like with our definition. We can use Fisher's definition and require that 95% of the evidence support our conclusion (a 5% error rate). In this case, the boundaries of our confidence interval will be set at 1.65 standard deviations (2 standard deviations would provide a boundary of 97.5%, remember?). To make things easier, a 1 standard deviation boundary provides a support level of 84% and a 1.5 standard deviation boundary provides a level of 93%. The boundary choice is up to you. I will use 95% boundaries (90% confidence intervals) for most of the examples in this book.

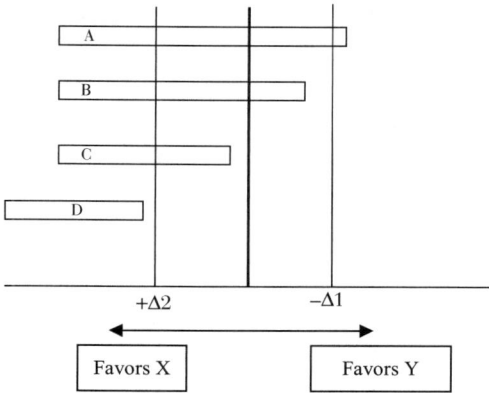

Figure 4-4. 90% Confidence intervals with 95% lower boundaries demonstrating possible outcomes of a clinical trial. A = indeterminate result due to inadequate sample size; B = X not inferior to Y ($p > .05$); C = X not inferior to Y ($p < .05$); D = X superior to Y ($p < .05$).

Now we can put things together. If we consider any clinical trial comparing drug X and drug Y, there are really only three possible outcomes: *(1)* one of the two drugs is superior to the other; *(2)* there is no difference between the two drugs; or *(3)* the study was too small and no conclusion can be drawn. Figure 4-4 shows four outcome scenarios for a clinical trial comparing drug X and drug Y. The dark line represents the line of indifference (1 in the case of likelihood or rate ratios). The vertical line $-\Delta 1$ represents one threshold of clinical significance, where we would consider Y superior (15%, for the sake of this discussion), and $+\Delta 2$ represents the other threshold of clinical significance, where we would consider X as superior. In the vast majority of cases the absolute value of $-\Delta 1 = +\Delta 2$. Bars A, B, C, and D represent the 90% confidence intervals for possible outcomes of the study.

Bar A shows that the lower limit is below the line of indifference and below the lower clinical threshold while the upper limit exceeds the upper clinical threshold. In this case we cannot draw any conclusion since the preponderance of evidence provides no support to any inference. This is an example of a study that is underpowered, that is, not enough subjects were included in the study and as a result the confidence interval is too broad to draw an inference.

Bar B shows that the lower limit of the 90% confidence interval is above the lower clinical threshold but below the line of indifference. In this example, we can state that the preponderance of evidence (95% in this case) is above the lower clinical threshold and we can infer that drug X is *not inferior* to drug Y. If the upper limit of Bar B was below $+\Delta 2$, we could infer, by convention, that drug X is *equivalent* to drug Y, although the clinical distinction between "not inferior" and "equivalent" is unclear.

Bar C shows that the lower limit of the 90% confidence interval is above the line of indifference but below $+\Delta 2$, the upper threshold for clinical significance. In traditional statistics this would suggest that that drug X is statistically superior to drug Y since 95% of the evidence is above the line of indifference. From the point of view of clinical significance, Bar C supports the same inference as Bar B, namely that drug X is not inferior to drug Y. For Bar D, the lower limit of the 90% confidence interval is greater than the upper threshold of clinical significance (15% in our example) and above the line of indifference. In this case we can state that the preponderance of evidence (95% of the data) exceeds the upper threshold of clinical significance, and we can infer that drug X is superior to drug Y. A mirror set of outcome intervals could be identified that would show that Y is not inferior, equivalent to, or superior to X.

The limitation of traditional error testing is clear from these examples. Lower boundary limits above the line of indifference occur in cases where there is no clinical difference between two therapies (or a new therapy and placebo) and in cases where a clinical difference exists. As a result, traditional statistical methods do not permit an assessment of clinical significance. We will use the method of preponderance of evidence along with other methods to answer questions in the following chapters.

5

ANSWERING A
QUESTION REGARDING
THE TREATMENT
OF A DISEASE

Developing an appropriate clinical question, searching the medical literature, and finding evidence are the initial steps in the medical decision-making process. Regardless of the type of question, the evidence must be validated before it can be analyzed for clinical significance. The validation criteria vary depending on the nature of the clinical question. In this section as in many of the other sections, the criteria for validation will be provided as a series of questions. Most of these validation criteria are adapted from Sackett et al.'s *Evidence Based Medicine: How to Practice and Teach EBM* (Churchill-Livingston, London, 2000) as well as *The Journal of the American Medical Association*'s *User's Guide to the Medical Literature* (McGraw-Hill, U.S.A., 2nd edition, 2008).

The criteria for validating a therapeutic study are well defined. In fact, the Food and Drug Administration (FDA) typically requires clinical trials that meet the following criteria to be completed before new agents can be licensed and released in the United States:

1. *Were the subjects well defined at the time of enrollment?* Patient status and diagnosis need to be homogeneous and clear in the subject groups. Inclusion and exclusion criteria need to be stated. It would be difficult to assess the results of a new bronchodilator if the patient population included children with cystic fibrosis and bronchopulmonary dysplasia as well as asthma. As noted earlier, it is also difficult to extend adult data to neonatal and infant patients.

2. *Was there an appropriate control group?* Modern experimental
   theory requires that outcomes for a new therapy be compared
   contemporaneously with outcomes from either standard therapy
   or placebo (no therapy). Given the possibilities of selection bias
   as well as changes in confounding variables (e.g., concomitant
   care), historical controls are largely unacceptable. Placebo control also permits successful blinding as to outcome. If standard
   therapy has been shown to have a benefit, it is unethical to use
   a placebo for comparison. For example, given the impact of
   combination therapy on the natural history of HIV infections,
   placebo-controlled trials of new agents would not be ethically or
   morally acceptable.
3. *Were patients effectively randomized to treatment or control?*
   Selection bias is a major problem with open, nonrandom-
   ized trials. If the investigator believes that the new therapy
   is better than the old, he is more likely to enroll the sickest
   patients in the treatment arm of the study. Randomization
   is undertaken to minimize the risk of unbalanced subgroups
   and to control for unforeseen covariates. In most studies, the
   investigator and the patient are blinded as to the assignment
   of the patient.

   Randomization is set up in advance and monitored by a
   third party. Often, randomization is performed in blocks; for
   example, in blocks of 10, 5 control and 5 treatment patients
   would be assigned for every 10 patients enrolled. Which of
   those patients were in which group would remain hidden.
4. *Was a relevant outcome selected?* The primary outcome selected
   for the trial should be clinically relevant. For example, the
   outcome selected for an asthma therapy trial may be length
   of hospitalization, intensive care unit admission rate, duration
   of intubation, or hospitalization rate (if an outpatient trial).
   Looking at oxygen saturation or a clinical score 2 hours after
   drug administration is unlikely to hold much sway. In many
   studies, a host of outcomes may be put forth in the Results
   section; however, each study needs to have a single, primary
   outcome.
5. *Were all patients accounted for at the conclusion of the study?*
   Many clinical trials require serial evaluations and drug admin-
   istrations over an extended period of time. As such, dropouts
   become a significant problem. False starts occur when a patient
   is enrolled, has received drug, and then is discovered to have
   failed to meet the inclusion criteria or has an exclusion criterion.
   All of the patients who were enrolled and received drug must be
   accounted for at the end of the trial.
6. *Was an intent to treat analysis performed?* All studies will
   include a per protocol analysis, that is, a comparison of

outcomes among patients who completed the investigational protocol. Each study should also compare primary outcomes in all patients enrolled, regardless of whether they completed the study. Requiring this degree of "robustness" for the results reduces confounding systematic bias. Moreover, keeping patients in their original groups, regardless of whether they completed their treatment, is consistent with the assumption that assignment to groups is random and that any treatment effect that appears is random. Removing patients from either group because of dropout or failure to adhere to the protocol runs the risk of introducing systematic bias and invalidating the study.

7. *Was the power of the study determined?* As you will recall from Chapter 4, under the Neyman–Pearson theory type I or α error is the probability that the data from the study will lead you to falsely accept the tested hypothesis, while type II or β error is the probability that the data from the study will lead you to falsely accept the alternative hypothesis. While the method of preponderance of evidence does not use these values, calculations of the power of a study provide a useful estimate of the sample size required for a successful study. Power $(1 - \beta)$ is a function of effect size (the difference in outcome rates between the treatment and the control group) and the outcome rate in the control group. For example, a large sample size is required if the difference in outcome rates between the treatment and the control group is 90%, but the prevalence of the outcome in the control group is only 1%. Adequate power (defined variably as .80 to .90) should lead to sufficiently narrow confidence intervals so that a clinical inference can be drawn (see Fig. 4-3). Narrowing the confidence interval will allow you to draw a clinical inference without altering the amount of evidence supporting your conclusion.

8. *Were the investigators and subjects blinded as to treatment assignment?* Modern clinical trials randomize patients to a treatment group and a comparison group (standard therapy or placebo). In a single-blinded study, these assignments are hidden from the subjects; in a double-blinded study these assignments are hidden from both the subjects and the investigators. Blinding is used in most clinical trials to avoid outcome bias. Patients (or investigators) who know that the subject has been randomized to receive the new treatment may "see" clinical improvement or drug side effects because of heightened expectations. The opposite is true for those randomized to standard therapy or placebo. Blinding is a way to keep the determination of each patient's outcome "honest."

STUDY DESIGN

Valid therapeutic studies are randomized clinical trials. As discussed previously, *parallel* studies require the concurrent enrollment of treatment and control patients, while *cross-over* studies use the same patients in both arms of the study. In cross-over studies, assignment as to which arm is first and which is last is determined randomly. The latter type of design requires fewer patients and has narrower variances since comparisons are paired (one comparison for each patient). Cross-over studies are limited by the possibility of drug carryover effect from one period to the next and by the natural progression of the disease process.

SUCCESS OF RANDOMIZATION

Simply because the patients were randomized to treatment and placebo groups does not ensure that the two groups are identical. Typically, the first table presented in the Results section of a randomized clinical trial compares the demography of the treatment and the control groups. Age, sex, disease state, and baseline measures should all be recorded. Differences between the groups may or may not invalidate the study. For example, a small difference in age may be of little consequence in an asthma study, while a significant difference in pulmonary function at the time of enrollment may invalidate the study results.

ASSESSMENT OF CLINICAL SIGNIFICANCE

The initial assessment of a clinical trial is determined by the preponderance of evidence, using the rate ratio for the primary outcome. In cases where no inference can be drawn or where an inference of not inferior or equivalence is made, the process stops. Nothing further can be learned from the data set. You may see arguments independent of the clinical significance made in the latter case. For example, if an inference of not inferior is made and drug X is substantially cheaper than drug Y, is easier to use, is more readily available, or has a superior safety profile to drug Y, you may choose to use drug X. Consider the following example:

> Reteplase is a tissue plaminogen activator with a longer half-life than alteplase, a drug that was used in the late 1990s to open blocked coronary arteries (*N Engl J Med* 1997; 337:1118–1123). A multicenter, randomized trial was undertaken to compare the two drugs and was powered ($1 - \beta$ to detect a 20% relative reduction in mortality at 30 days of follow-up. The mortality rates for the reteplase and alteplase groups were .0747 (757/10,138) and .0724 (356/4921), respectively.

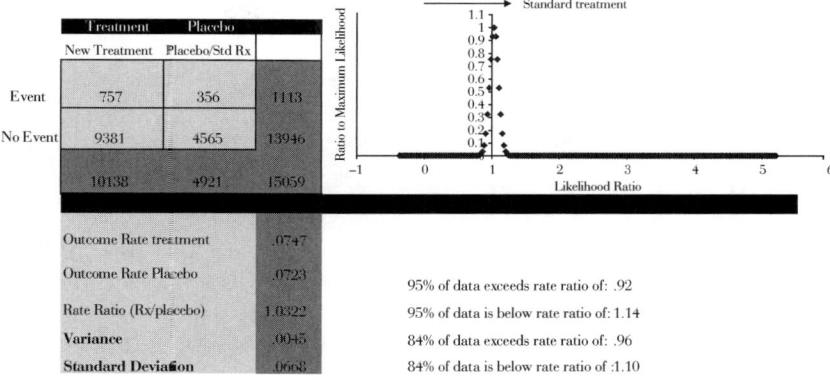

Figure 5-1. Likelihood probability function of reteplase (new treatment) vs. alteplase (Std RX) for the prevention of death following coronary events. Lower 95% boundary = .92 (no more than 8% increased risk with alteplase); upper 95% boundary = 1.14 (no more than 14% increase risk with reteplase). Lower 84% boundary = .96 (no more than 4% increased risk with alteplase); upper 84% boundary = 1.10 (no more than 105 increased risk with reteplase). (From GUSTO III Investigators. A Comparison of retaplase with alteplase for acute myocardial infarction. *N Engl J Med* 1997; 337:1118–1123.)

These rates were entered into a simple Excel-based program and the results are shown in Figure 5-1. Overall, the death rate ratio was 1.03, 3% higher in the treatment (reteplase) group. Using the preponderance of evidence method, we can state that 95% of the data supports a mortality rate in the alteplase group that exceeds the rate in the reteplase group by no more than 8% (1 – .92), and 84% of the data supports a mortality rate in the alteplase group that exceeds the rate in the reteplase group by no more than 4% (1 – .96). You can also see that reteplase is no more than 10% (1.10 – 1) to 14% (1.14 – 1) worse than alteplase with regard to mortality. It is therefore reasonable to conclude that the two drugs are therapeutically equivalent. Since the safety profiles were similar and since reteplase is easier to administer, an argument could be made for the superiority of reteplase on grounds other than clinical efficacy. The huge size of this trial was required due to the low mortality rate in the alteplase (standard therapy) group; otherwise the confidence intervals would have been too large to draw any inference.

As noted earlier, outcomes may be expressed as *rate ratios, odds ratios,* or *rate differences. Relative risk reduction* is typically used in vaccine trials. There are some advantages in the way outcomes are expressed. Consider the following example:

A vaccine is developed for a common respiratory virus of childhood. A large, multicenter, randomized, double-blinded, placebo-controlled was completed. The primary endpoint for the study was infection. The following data were obtained:

	Infected	Noninfected	Total
Vaccine	100	9900	10,000
Control	1000	9000	10,000

The infection rates for the vaccinees and controls are .01 (100/10,000) and .1 (1000/10,000), respectively. The *rate ratio* (control/vaccine) is 10; the *rate difference or absolute risk reduction* (control − vaccine) is .09; the *odds ratio* (control/vaccine) is 11 (9900 × 1000)/(9000 × 100); and the *vaccine efficacy rate (relative risk reduction)* is (.1 − .01)/.1 = .9. The data were also analyzed for hospitalization rates:

	Hospitalized	Not Hospitalized	Total
Vaccine	1	9999	10,000
Control	10	9990	10,000

The hospitalization rates for the vaccinees and controls are .0001 and .001, respectively. The *rate ratio* (control/vaccine) is 10, the *odds ratio* (control/vaccine) is 11, and the *vaccine efficacy rate* is .9. Despite a huge decrease in event rates, these outcome measures are unchanged! This failure to account for changes in control occurrence rate is a limitation to the use of these rates as the only measures of clinical significance.

What happened to the *rate difference*? The infection rate difference is .09 and the hospitalization rate difference is .0009. The rate difference reflects the changes in the underlying rate in the control group. Unfortunately, these values are not intuitively useful. The *number of patients who need to be treated* (NNT) in order to prevent an additional occurrence of the outcome event is defined by the reciprocal of the rate difference. Therefore, for infection, NNT = 1/.09 = 11 and for hospitalization NNT= 1/.0009 = 1111. In other words, on average 11 children need to be vaccinated to prevent one episode of infection and 1111 children need to be vaccinated to prevent a single hospitalization. Combined with the likelihood ratio, the rate difference provides an additional measure of clinical significance in clinical therapeutic trials. Let's look at another example:

> At the beginning of the AIDS epidemic in the United States, infants born to HIV-positive mothers were at significant risk for acquiring the infection. A large multicenter study randomized HIV-positive women to receive zidovudine (AZT) prior to delivery and during delivery and for their infants to receive AZT for the first 6 weeks of life; the comparison group of maternal–infant pairs

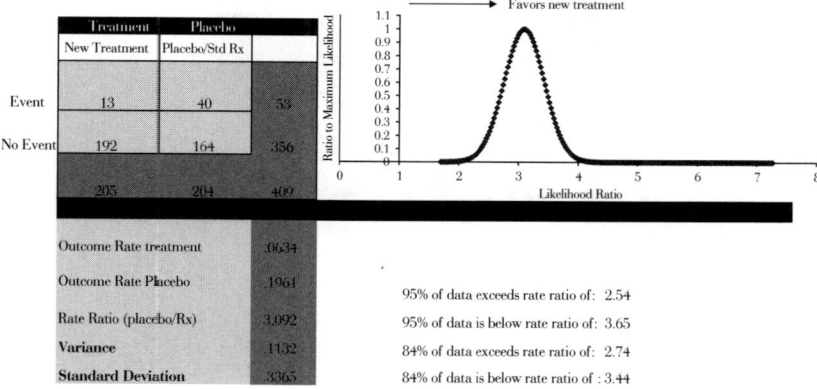

Figure 5-2. Incidence of neonatal human immunodeficiency virus infection in mother–infant pairs treated with zidovudine(AZT) or placebo. Lower 95% boundary = 2.54 (at least a 2.5-fold increased risk in placebo recipients); lower 84% boundary = 2.74 (at least a 2.7-fold increased risk in placebo recipients). (From Connor EM, et al. Reduction of maternal-infant transmission of human immunodeficiency virus type 1 with zidovudine treatment. *N Engl J Med* 1994; 331:1173–1180.)

received placebo medication on the same schedule. (*N Engl J Med* 1994; 331:1173–1180)

The primary outcome measure was the cumulative rate of HIV infection in the infants by 72 weeks of age. The infant infection rates were 19.6% (40/204) for the placebo recipients and 6.3% (13/205) for the AZT-treated group.

The results are shown in Figure 5-2. From the curve, it is clear that the infection rate among placebo recipients is statistically higher than the treated group, since 1 is nowhere near the curve. We can state that 95% of the data supports an infection rate in the placebo group that is at least 2.5 times higher than that in the treated group and that 84% of the data supports a placebo infection rate that is at least 2.7 times higher than the treated group. Clearly we can infer that AZT therapy is clinically significant. Using the rate ratios of .20 and .06 for the placebo and AZT groups, respectively, we find a rate difference of .14. Therefore, we can infer that, *on average*, for every 7 (1/.14) mother–infant pairs treated with AZT, one infant infection with HIV will be avoided. You can see why this was such a convincing study and why AZT therapy became the standard of care for HIV-infected mothers who are about to deliver.

Let's return to our first example that compared the efficacy of reteplase and alteplase. The absolute risk reduction = .074 – .072 = .02, favoring alteplase. The finding that *on average* 500 patients need to receive alteplase to avoid 1 death that would have occurred if reteplase had been used instead further underscores the clinical equivalence of the two drugs.

6

ANSWERING A QUESTION REGARDING THE UTILITY OF A DIAGNOSTIC TEST

When you consider the questions that patients ask physicians, "What's wrong with me?" is clearly the most fundamental. Without a diagnosis, issues of therapy, prognosis, and etiology cannot be addressed. A common misconception among both the lay public and physicians is that all diagnostic tests are definitive and that all tests have "bright line" cutoffs. While it is true that gold standards exist for many diagnoses (such as blood culture results for the diagnosis of bacteremia and biopsies for cancer), many tests with high degrees of precision ultimately prove unreliable in cases where the incidence of the disease in question is low.

VALIDATION

Studies that address issues of diagnosis need to meet several criteria in order for their results to be *valid*. The following are adapted from Sackett et al., *Clinical Epidemiology: A Basic Science for Clinical Medicine* (Boston: Little, Brown and Company, 2nd edition, 1991, p. 52):

1. *Has the diagnostic test been evaluated in an appropriate patient sample?* For these studies to be externally valid, a well-defined cohort of patients must be assembled at the onset of the study. The best studies are prospective and observational; retrospective studies using data gathered in databases or from hospital records are useful but less valid. The subjects should represent a sample of age-appropriate patients with the constellation of

clinical signs and symptoms of interest. For example, if your patient is a 14-year-old female with right-sided abdominal pain and a question of appendicitis, the results of a study of appendicitis in adults may not be valid. Age becomes an even bigger issue in neonates and young infants. Caution must be taken when applying adult data to children. It is also important to keep the sex and clinical setting of the patient in mind. The differential diagnosis of acute abdominal pain is different in females than males. Given the earlier example, it is reasonable to expect that the incidence of appendicitis would be higher if all of the patients were recruited from the office of a pediatric surgeon rather than the office of a general pediatrician or family physician. The incidence of gynecologic-related disorders would be higher if the patients were recruited from an adolescent or student health clinic.

2. *Has each patient in the cohort been evaluated by both the gold standard test and the test in question?* Within the assembled cohort of patients, two subgroups should emerge based on the results of the gold standard test: those patients with the disorder in question and those without it. It is only by comparing the results of the test in question between these defined subgroups that the precision of the test can be determined. In cases where the test in question requires subjective interpretation (such as imaging studies), the interpreter should be blinded to the diagnosis as determined by the gold standard. Sometimes no readily available gold standard exists. Kawasaki disease is a syndrome defined by an array of clinical findings that are not unique. Finally you can ask whether the management of the patient has changed as a result of the diagnostic test. Certainly this is the acid test for any standard of diagnosis.

3. *Does the cohort include patients with diseases that may be confused with the target disorder?* As the patients in the cohort are defined by the gold standard for the target disorder, representative patients with other, possibly confusing, disorders should be included. For example, a study of adolescents with right-sided abdominal pain could use the pathology of the appendix as the gold standard for appendicitis and abdominal ultrasound as the test in question. In the case of the 14-year-old female cited earlier, it is reasonable to expect patients with pelvic inflammatory disease and tubal pregnancies to be included in the cohort. Certainly you want to know whether abdominal ultrasonography could distinguish among these entities.

4. *Has the reproducibility of the test results and its interobservational variation been determined?* In tests where the result is based on observer interpretation (e.g., imaging tests, scoring of histologic findings, etc.), it is critical to know if separate observers came

to similar conclusions about the same test. Studies of this type need to include multiple observers looking at each test. A kappa measure of interobserver variability must be provided as part of the results.

5. *Have all of the terms used in the study been defined?* "Normal," "positive," and "negative" are terms that we all use when we discuss diagnostic tests. It is important that these terms be defined in the study. Returning to the case of our 14-year-old female with abdominal pain, it is important to know if a "negative" ultrasound study means that the appendix appeared to be normal to the observer or if it means that the observer was unable to see the appendix; the implications of each of these definitions are different.

6. *If the test is part of a series of tests, has its contribution to the series been determined?* Returning to our adolescent patient, suppose the diagnostic scheme of abdominal ultrasound followed by helical computed tomography (CT) with rectal contrast if the ultrasound is negative is proposed. Does the ultrasound offer any advantage over CT scans for all comers? Does a positive ultrasound require confirmation by CT scan? These questions must be answered in the context of the study.

PROPERTIES OF DIAGNOSTIC TESTS

Once you have determined that a study meets the validity criteria, you need to determine whether the study has value and what its utility is. The results of most studies that define a diagnostic test produce dichotomous results and can fit into a 2 × 2 table as seen in Figure 6-1.

All of the parameters of interest can be expressed in terms of a, b, c, and d as shown in Figure 6-1. The *prevalence* of the target disorder

| | Gold Standard | |
	Positive	Negative
Test Positive	a	b
Negative	c	d

Figure 6-1. 2 × 2 Box to determine the utility of a diagnostic test. Gold standard defines patients with target disorder. Test defines results of diagnostic test of interest. (See text for definitions of sensitivity, specificity, true and false positives, and true and false negatives, and positive and negative predictive values.)

in this population is defined as the proportion of subjects with the disorder in the total sample population. In this case the prevalence is equal to (a + c)/(a + b + c + d), since a + c equals all of the patients with the target disorder defined by the gold standard. The *sensitivity* or *true-positive rate* of the test is defined as the proportion of subjects with a positive test among the subpopulation of individuals with the target disorder: a/(a + c). Equally important, the *false-negative rate (FNR)* of the test is defined as the proportion of subjects with a negative test among the subpopulation of individuals *with* the target disorder: c/(a + c). The *specificity* or *true-negative rate* of the test is defined as the proportion of subjects with a negative test among the subpopulation of individuals free of the target disorder: d/(b + d). It should follow, therefore, that the *false-positive rate* of the test is the proportion of subjects with a positive test among those without the disorder: b/(b + d). Please note that 1 – specificity = false-positive rate and 1 – sensitivity = false-negative rate.

Given these relationships and assuming the test is positive, what conclusion can you draw regarding a test with a very high sensitivity (>95%)? Is this type of test useful for screening patients with a suspected disorder? Normally you would think that if a test has a 95% true-positive rate, then a positive test would rule in the target disorder. Unfortunately, the left-hand side of the 2 × 2 box gives you no information regarding the *false-positive* rate; it could be 90% without affecting the sensitivity of the test. You do know, however, that if the true-positive rate is very high, then the false-negative rate is very low (1 – sensitivity = false-negative rate)! *Thus, if a test with a high sensitivity is negative, you can rule out the target disorder.* Sackett et al. use the acronym SnNout to convey this concept. Any test that is a bona fide SnNout is a good screening test since it will effectively exclude a subpopulation from further evaluation.

Assuming that the test is negative, what conclusion can you draw regarding a test with a high specificity (95%)? Is this type of test useful for screening patients at risk for the target disorder? Similar to the previous discussion, the true-negative rate gives no information regarding the false-negative rate; that information is contained in the sensitivity of the test. Specificity does include a measure of the false-positive rate and it follows that for *tests with high specificity, a positive result will rule in the target disorder.* Sackett et al. use the acronym SpPin to convey this concept. Any test that is a bona fide SpPin can establish the disease if it is positive. Keep in mind that if the test does not also have a very high sensitivity, then a negative test does *not* exclude the target disorder.

While sensitivity and specificity are useful concepts for remembering the strengths and weaknesses of a given test for a specific target disease, what you really want to know is the predictive value of a positive and negative test; that is, if a test is positive, what is the likelihood that patients have the target disorder, and if the test is negative, what is the likelihood that they do not. The *positive predictive value* (PPV) is defined as the probability of a patient with a positive test having the target disorder. Using the 2 × 2 box in Figure 6-1, the PPV is a/(a + b). The *negative predictive value* (NPV) is defined similarly and is given by the expression d/(c + d). The positive and negative predictive values of a gold standard test should approach 100%. One measure of the predictive value of a test is its *accuracy*, defined as the (sensitivity + specificity)/2. This metric, however, does not provide a useful construct for calculating predictive values.

BAYES THEORUM

The positive and negative predictive values have an interesting property. Assume that a given test has a sensitivity of 95% and a specificity of 92%. Also assume that the prevalence of the target disorder is 30%. For 1000 patients, the 2 × 2 table shown in Figure 6-2 would apply. In this case, the positive predictive value is around 84% and the negative predictive value is about 98%. What happens if we shift to a population where the prevalence is only 2% (Fig. 6-3)? Without changing the sensitivity or the specificity of the test, the positive predictive value has fallen to 20% and the negative predictive value has increased to almost 100%. Does this suggest a way that data can influence your thinking about the probability of an event?

The dual phenomena of increasing negative predictive value and decreasing positive predictive value with decreasing prevalence is predicted by Bayes theorum. Bayesian statistics permit the translation of the prevalence rate into the positive or negative predictive value using a Bayesian factor that is dependent exclusively on the test characteristics. Since the Bayesian factor is expressed as a likelihood ratio (true rate/false rate) exactly as the outcomes of a clinical trial are expressed, we have to express the prevalence of the disorder in the sample population in a similar way. If the prevalence rate is .30 in our population, then the likelihood ratio of having the disease is the rate of those with the disease divided by the rate of those

	Gold Standard			
	Positive	Negative	Total	
Positive	285	56	341	.84 **Positive Predictive Value**
Test				
Negative	15	644	659	.98 **Negative Predictive Value**
Total	300	700		
Sensitivity	.95	.92	**Specificity**	
			Prevalence	.30

Figure 6-2. Bayes theorem I. Determination of positive and negative predictive values when test characteristics are fixed (sensitivity = .95; specificity = .92) and prevalence rate of target disorder is 30% (.30).

| | Gold Standard | | | |
	Positive	Negative	Total	
Positive	19	78.4	97.4	0.20 **Positive Predictive Value**
Test				
Negative	1	901.6	902.6	1.00 **Negative Predictive Value**
Total	20	980		
Sensitivity	.95	.92	**Specificity**	
			Prevalence	.02

Figure 6-3. Bayes theorem II. Determination of positive and negative predictive values when test characteristics are fixed (sensitivity = .95; specificity = .92) and prevalence rate of target disorder is 2% (.02).

without the disease. In this case, the a priori likelihood ratio defining the prevalence of the disease for our sample population is $.30/(1 - .30)$ or .43. *The pretest probability, or prevalence rate, p, can be converted to the a priori odds or likelihood ratio, Po, by the formula $Po = p/(1 - p)$.*

The *Bayesian factor* for a test designed to increase the a priori odds is called the *positive likelihood ratio*. In this case, a positive test result increases the likelihood of the target disorder and the positive likelihood ratio must be greater than 1. For any diagnostic test, the positive likelihood ratio is the true-positive rate (sensitivity) divided by the false-positive rate (1 – specificity). For our example, the positive likelihood ratio is $.95/(1 - .92) = 11.9$.

Bayes theorum contends that:

$$A \ priori \ odds \times Bayes \ factor = Posterior \ (post \ test) \ odds$$

Thus, $.43 \times 11.9 = 5.12$. *The posterior odds, Op, can be converted to the posterior probability or predictive value, p′, by the simple formula: $p′ = Op/(1 + Op)$.* In this case, $p′ = 5.12/(1 + 5.12) = .84$. In our example, then, the probability that a patient with a positive test has the target disorder is 84% if the prevalence rate of the target disorder in the patient population is 30%. Using the same positive likelihood ratio, we can calculate that the posterior odds of the target disorder when the a priori odds are .0204 (a priori probability = 2%) is .24. Converting this to a probability we get 19.5%.

Look at the huge impact prevalence has on the posterior odds. Notice that the characteristics of the test, as defined by the positive likelihood ratio, did not change. Also notice that the posterior odds, when converted to probabilities, are equal to the positive predictive values calculated from the 2 × 2 tables!

We can use Bayes theorum to calculate the negative predictive value as well. Remember that the a priori odds were defined as $p/1 - p$, where p was the prevalence rate. Since $1 - p$ is the probability that patients do *not* have the target disorder, then the reciprocal of the a priori odds, $(1 - p)/p$, is the initial odds that patients do not have the disease. In the earlier example, the rate ratio of *no* disease = .7/.3 *or* 1/.43 or 2.33. The *negative likelihood ratio* is the Bayesian factor that will increase this value and it is defined as the ratio of the true-negative rate to the false-negative rate (specificity/(1 –sensitivity). For the example, the negative likelihood ratio is $.92/(1 - .95) = 18.4$ and the posterior odds are 42.9 (2.33×18.4). The negative predictive value is 97.7%, identical to that calculated in Figure 6-2. Notice that this test is a stronger negative predictor than positive predictor since the positive likelihood ratio is only 11.9.

Finally, Bayes theorum permits the "stringing together" of diagnostic tests. If a patient has X positive tests and the characteristics of all of the tests are defined by positive likelihood ratios $(LR_1, LR_2...LR_x)$, then the posterior odds are defined as: a priori odds $\times (LR_1 \times LR_2 \times ...LR_x)$. This property of Bayes theorum forms the basis for the clinical prediction rules that we will discuss later.

Let's look at an interesting example of how the test characteristics and the prevalence of disease in the sample population influence predictive values. In 2009, infection with the novel influenza strain H1N1 was widespread in the United States. In the spring and fall of that year, testing for the disease using rapid antigen detection assays was largely discouraged by the Centers for Disease Control and Prevention. When I asked students and residents on rounds why this was so, the uniform response was that the sensitivity of the test was poor and therefore it was not a useful test to screen for influenza. When we looked for evidence to support this, several studies were found. The most applicable to our population of children was: Uyeki T, et al. Low sensitivity of rapid diagnostic test for influenza. *Clin Infect Dis* 2009; 48:e89. In this study, the authors determined the sensitivity and specificity of a rapid influenza test using a nucleic acid detection test (RT-PCR) as the gold standard. Over 600 college students and children were recruited at three sites. Over the course of the study, 47% of the enrollees were PCR positive for influenza. From the data provided in the paper, the following summative properties of the test were calculated: Sensitivity (true-positive rate) = .25; Specificity (true-negative rate) = .98; positive likelihood ratio = 12.5; negative likelihood ratio = 1.3. Converting the incidence to odds, $.47/(1 - .47) = .89$, we can calculate the positive (PPV) and negative predictive values (NPV) for this study:

$$PPV = .89 \times 12.5 = 11.1$$
$$NPV = (1/.89) \times 1.3 = 1.5$$

Converting odds to probabilities, we find that the PPV is .92 while the negative predictive value is only .6. These data support the students' contention that the rapid test is a poor screening test, since 40% of patients with a negative test may be infected. Conversely, this is a good confirmatory test, since patients with a positive test are very likely (92%) to actually have the disease (low false-positive rate). So the students and residents were right...or were they?

Consider a normal summer when the incidence of influenza among children with fever and cough is approximately 5%. How useful is this test in the summertime to screen for influenza? Let's see:

$$PPV = (.05/.95) \times 12.5 = .66$$
$$NPV = (.95/.05) \times 1.3 = 24.7$$

Converting back to probabilities we find that the PPV is only .4 while the negative predictive value is .96. So, in the summertime, a child with fever and cough and a negative rapid influenza test almost certainly does not have the flu (4% error rate), However, a child with the same symptoms and a positive test has a 60% chance of not having the flu but instead has a false-positive test. While the test characteristics have not changed, the utility of the test has changed dramatically. The rapid test is a poor screening test during epidemics of influenza but is a useful confirmatory test for the disease, while the exact opposite is true in the off season. So what answer can we offer the student or resident who asks about the utility of the test? It depends.

RECEIVER–OPERATOR CURVES

In many studies of diagnostic tests, the tests under scrutiny may have a range of values. Antibody titers and acute reactants such as serum concentrations of C-reactive protein, IL-6, procalcitonin, and erythrocyte sedimentation rates are examples of tests used to predict the outcome of gold standard tests such as cultures, nucleic acid amplification, biopsies, or invasive imaging. In general, low concentrations of these serum tests will be sensitive (high true-positive rates) but not specific (low true-negative rates). At very high concentrations, the opposite is true. How do we find the best cutoff value for these tests?

A similar problem existed during World War II with the use of radar. At very high frequencies, the returning signals were strong, but the output of the original sets included a lot of artifact (high sensitivity/low specificity). When lower frequencies were used, many enemy aircraft were missed (high specificity/low sensitivity). The solution was to maximize the signal-to-noise ratio by using plots of true-positive rates versus false-positive rates. Consider Figure 6-4. The dotted line represents the *line of indifference*. Points along this line cannot discriminate true from false. The other two lines represent two separate tests and were generated from a single data set; different cutoff points were used to make a dichotomous outcome determination (e.g., disease or no disease; cure or failure). In essence, each point on a line would represent a different 2 × 2 box generated from a different cutoff value. The lower solid line shows a test with some discriminatory power; the upper solid line shows a better test. The probability that a test will discriminate correctly between outcomes is approximated by the area under the curve. The best cutoff value is that

Table 6-1.   Comparison of True-Positive and False-Positive Rates of Urine White Blood Cell Counts in Patients with Clinical Symptoms of Urinary Tract Infections

White Blood Cells (Cells/mm³)	True-Positive Rate (%)	False-Positive Rate (%)
15	89	2.4
10	91	3.4
5	96	13

Source. Reprinted with permission from Hoberman, et al. Pyuria and bacteriuria in urine specimens obtained by catheter from young children with fever. *J Pediatr.* 1994; 124:513–519.

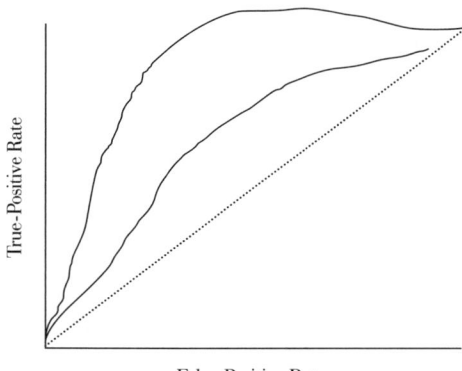

False-Positive Rate

Figure 6-4.   Receiver–operator curve. Results of two different diagnostic tests. Dotted line is line of indifference.

point on the curve closest to the left upper corner, where the true-positive rate/false-positive rate is the greatest.

Let's look at an example. Hoberman et al. wanted to determine the cutoff value of white blood cells in the urine from young infants that would strongly predict a positive urine culture of >50,000 CFU/mL (*J Pediatr* 1994; 124:513). Samples were collected from 2181 children less than 2 years of age; three cell count values were examined in detail (Table 6-1). The positive likelihood ratios (TPR/FPR) for 15, 10, and 5 cells/mm³ were 37, 26, and 7.4, respectively. Which value would you select as a bright line cutoff? Although the authors chose 10 cells/mm³ because of the slightly higher true-positive rate and the "comparable" false-positive rate, 15 cells/mm³ produces a higher positive likelihood ratio. In this study, the prevalence rate of urine cultures with >50,000 CFU/mL was 4.2% (a priori odds = .044). Using 15 cells/mm³ and 10 cells/mm³ as cutoff points, the posterior odds are 1.62 (PPV = 62%) and 1.14 (PPV = 53%), respectively, suggesting that 15 cells/mm³ is a better positive predictor.

UNCERTAINTY AND DIAGNOSTIC TESTS

Up to this point, all of the discussion and applications have focused on the central value of the positive or the negative predictive value. Since all of these values are derived from experimental samples, some degree of uncertainty must exist around these values. As it turns out, it is easy to apply the preponderance of evidence principle to simple diagnostic tests. In the previous example, given a urinary tract infection prevalence rate of .042, the positive prediction values were .62 and .53 when children had 15 or 10 cells/mm^3 in the urine, respectively. For reasons not worth going into here, we will use the standard error in place of the standard deviation in order to apply the principle of the preponderance of evidence. For a simple proportion, p, and subject size, n, the standard error is defined as $\sqrt{p(1-p)/n}$. Therefore, for a cutoff of 15 cells/mm^3, the standard error is $\sqrt{.62 \times .38/2181}$ or .01; for 10 cells/mm^3, the standard error is $\sqrt{.53 \times .47/n}$ or .005. Assuming a prevalence rate of .04 and using 1.65 standard error to determine the 95% lower confidence limit, we can state that for 15 cells/mm^3, 95% of the data supports a positive predictive value of .60 or greater and for 10 cells/mm^3, 95% of the data supports a positive predictive value of .52 or greater. The 84% lower confidence limits (–1 standard error) would be .61 and .52 for 15 cells/mm^3 and 10 cells/mm^3, respectively.

When using diagnostic tests, keep in mind that the utility of the test lies in its positive or negative predictive value. Both of these values are dependent on the characteristics of the test (likelihood ratio) *and* the prevalence of the disease in the population of interest (a priori odds). In the previous example where we examined white blood cell counts in urine to predict positive urine cultures, a 4.2% prevalence rate was in a general population of children under 2 years of age. In a population of sexually active adult women, the prevalence rate of urinary tract infections would be much higher, producing a larger positive predictive value. In a population of circumcised males under 2 years of age, the prevalence of urinary tract infections would likely be much less than 4.2%, producing a much lower positive predictive value. In any case, it is essential to determine whether the patient population that was used to generate the data is similar to the patient you have in the office, clinic, emergency department, or hospital.

7

ANSWERING A QUESTION REGARDING PROGNOSIS AND RISK FACTORS

After a diagnosis is made, the likely outcome of the disease process needs to be determined. Many diseases are self-limited. Other diseases, such as bacterial meningitis, despite prompt and aggressive therapy leave patients with residual disabilities or result in death. Consider the following case:

> A 10-month-old female infant presents to the emergency room following her first seizure. Her mother states that she was well until 2 days ago when she developed rhinorrhea, cough, and fever to 102°F. About an hour ago the child became unresponsive and developed generalized "twitching." Upon presentation to the emergency room, the child was febrile and unarousable. Her blood pressure was low, her extremities were cold, and her pulse was high. A lumbar puncture was consistent with bacterial meningitis. She was admitted to the intensive care unit and started on antibiotics, given intravenous fluids and ventilated. After 72 hours the child was still having seizures. The mother asks you what her likely outcome is.

What do you tell this child's mother? What is the likelihood of death, severe mental retardation, or epilepsy (afebrile seizures)? What additional data would help you answer these questions? To answer questions of prognosis, a valid study needs to meet a number of criteria:

1. *Was a cohort of patients assembled early in the course of the disease?* To be valid, these studies need to be performed forward in time. Examinations of large databases are less valid. In the case

of the child with bacterial meningitis, identifying children at a time beyond their initial presentation rather than at the time of their illness may bias the data for the following reasons: *(1)* a child with severe bacterial disease is more likely to be enrolled in the study than a child with mild disease, since the mild disease may be missed or not referred for admission (selection bias); *(2)* the specifics of the neurological status prior to the onset of disease are less likely to be recalled accurately at a time removed from the event (recall bias); *(3)* there is a significant mortality at presentation, those patients may be missed or the mortality rate may be underestimated and; *(4)* finally enrollment of consecutive patients is preferred to further eliminate selection bias.

2. *Do the patients represent population-based samples?* Although we require valid prognosis studies to assemble a cohort, the source of that cohort is important. Consider the case just described. Would the prognosis vary if we selected a sample of children who were seen in a pediatrician's office as opposed to a sample who were seen in an emergency room? Would the outcome differ if we selected a sample from the emergency room of a rural community hospital as opposed to a sample from a busy, urban pediatric emergency room? Which of these outcomes would be correct? Obviously, the best answer would be a sample selected from the general population, for example, all children born in the United States in a given year. When considering the applicability of prognostic data, consider the differences and similarities between your setting and the setting described in the study.

3. *Was the outcome for the study well defined and was follow-up adequate?* For a prognostic study to be meaningful, the outcome needs to be meaningful. For example, a 1-year follow-up of developmental achievement in a cohort of children with meningitis would not be useful in addressing the issue of long-term school performance. Similarly, the occurrence rate of afebrile seizures 6 months after the presentation would add little to the prognosis for lifelong epilepsy in this patient population. In most studies, you will see the use of survival curves to predict the occurrence rates of adverse outcomes long into the future. This type of data is used to determine which subgroups have an increased risk for bad outcomes and to shorten the length of follow-up needed.

4. *Were patients stratified according to risk?* Outcome analysis should be performed for subgroups with different prognostic factors. In the case of our example, patients should be stratified based on bacterial isolate, presence or absence of seizures, and presence or absence of shock. Individual survival curves should be developed for each subgroup.

With these criteria in mind, let's see what the evidence has to say about the prognosis of bacterial meningitis in children.

LITERATURE SEARCH

The clinical queries search engine of PubMed was used. The search string was "bacterial meningitis" AND children AND "risk factors"; a narrow search was chosen. This search yielded 39 results; one article will be discussed in detail.

The Evidence: J Paediatr Child Health *1996; 32:457*

This study identified a cohort of 166 children with bacterial meningitis diagnosed in the 1983–1986 timeframe. Most of the patients (133) were reevaluated between 1991 and 1993. Following reevaluation, the children were assigned to one of three outcome groups: normal, minor adverse outcomes (marginal IQ scores, mild to moderate hearing loss, or inability to read by age 7), and major adverse outcomes (death or severe intellectual, neurological, or audiological deficits). In the end, 95 (69%), 24 (18%), and 19 (14%) of the subjects had no, minor, or major adverse outcomes, respectively.

In many studies of this type, a *univariate analysis* is the first attempt to identify risk factors that will segregate patients into different outcome categories. In brief, the rate ratios for each potential risk factor are calculated and the dreaded p values are determined (see Chapter 4). In these types of studies, the p value helps to identify those factors with the greatest potential to differentiate outcome states. In this study, six such factors were identified with p values $<.05$: age <12 months at presentation, seizures in hospital, seizures 72 hours after treatment, return to normal mental status by 72 hours, deteriorating state of consciousness, cerebrospinal fluid leukocytes <1000 cells/mm^3, and serum sodium <130 mmol/L. The presence of any of these risk factors, except return to normal status by 72 hours, was associated with a higher risk for an adverse outcome; normalization of mental status was associated with an improved outcome.

The authors could stop here, but most do not and should not. This simple compilation of risk factors does not differentiate dependent variables from independent variables. *Dependent variables* (also known as response variables) represent an outcome. The *independent variables* represent the risk factors that cause the different outcomes. Using a statistical process called logistic regression, dependent variables can be separated from the independent variables or risk factors. In this study, age <12 months, deteriorating mental status, and seizures >72 hours after treatment were associated with major adverse outcomes.

How can we apply these data to the clinical situation? If we think of each risk factor as a diagnostic test for the "gold standard" (major adverse outcomes), we can use the same method for determining risk that we used for determining diagnostic utility. Table 7-1 shows the sensitivity,

Table 7-1. Risk Factors Associated with Severe Outcomes in Childhood
Bacterial Meningitis

Risk Factor	Sensitivity	Specifity	+LR
<12 Months of age	0.63	0.66	1.83
Deteriorating mental state	0.68	0.86	4.79
Seizures after 72 hours	0.42	0.97	12.53

Source. Reprinted with permission from Grimwood K, et al. Risk factors for adverse outcomes of
bacterial meningitis. *J Pediatr Child Health.* 1996; 32:457–462.

specificity, and positive likelihood ratio for each of the three risk factors
identified in the study. From the data in the paper we know that the
prevalence rate of major adverse outcomes is 14% (a priori odds = .16).
Therefore, for infants less than 12 months of age, the average *odds* of
a major adverse outcome are given by the equation: .16 × 1.83 = .29.
Converting odds to probability, the **AVERAGE RISK PROBABILITY**
that a child less than 12 months of age will suffer a major adverse outcome
is .23. Repeat this process and convince yourself that the average risk
probabilities of a major adverse outcome for children with deteriorating
mental status or seizures after 72 hours are .44 and .67, respectively.

As was the case with issues of diagnosis and therapy, there is uncertainty in ascribing risk to patients based on the presence or absence of
specific risk factors. Fortunately, the methods used in prognosis are identical to those used in diagnosis. In the case of prognosis, however, we are
interested in defining the risk by its maximum probability. To assess the
risk of a major adverse outcome for a child with bacterial meningitis by
using the same method discussed in Chapter 6, the associated standard
errors are .036, .04, and .043 and the 90% upper confidence limits are
.35, .50, and .74 for infants less than 12 months of age, with deteriorating mental status or with seizures after 72 hours, respectively. In the
absence of any risk factors, 95% of the evidence supports a risk of no more
than 19% that a child with bacterial meningitis will suffer a major adverse
event; the average risk for these children is 14%. For a child less than 12
months of age with bacterial meningitis, 95% of the evidence supports a
risk of no more than 35% with an average risk of a major adverse event of
23%. For a child with bacterial meningitis and deteriorating mental status
during hospitalization, 95% of the evidence supports a risk of no more
than 50% and an average risk of 44%. For a child with bacterial meningitis
and seizures that continue beyond 72 hours, 95% of the evidence supports
a risk of no more than 74% and an average risk of 67% for the occurrence
of a major adverse outcome.

As with diagnostic tests, risk factors can be combined using Bayes
theorem. For the patient in the example who is both less than 12 months
of age and has continuing seizures at 72 hours, the posterior odds of a
major adverse outcome are defined by the following: .16 × 1.83 × 12.53;
converting the resultant odds to probability yields an *average* risk of

79% for a major adverse outcome. Combining risk factors is the first step toward developing a clinical prediction rule. We will examine this in more detail in the next chapter.

In practice, take care that the precision of the mathematics does not lull you into a false sense of certainty with regard to prediction of clinical outcomes. These techniques do not provide a "crystal ball" for seeing into the future. Sometimes it is difficult to communicate this to the family. One approach is to use language to describe ranges of risk. Where the maximum estimated risk is less than 20%, we could state that there is a risk of a serious adverse event. When the maximum risk is less than 40%, we could say to this child's family that there is *some* risk of a serious adverse event. When the maximum risk is less than 60%, we could say to this child's family that there is a *substantial* risk of a serious adverse event. And when the maximum risk exceeds 60%, we could say that there is a *great* risk of a serious adverse event.

8

ANSWERING A
QUESTION USING A
CLINICAL PREDICTION
RULE

Clinical prediction rules may be applied to questions of diagnosis or prognosis, since rules may predict the results of a "gold standard" diagnostic test or the likelihood of a significant clinical event. One of the earliest examples of clinical prediction rules came from the Framingham Heart Study (http://www.framinghamheartstudy.org) that began in 1948; its risk profiles continue to be clinically useful today.

The usefulness of these rules is derived directly from Bayes theorem:

(1) A priori odds × likelihood ratio = posterior odds

The *a priori odds* are a restatement of the prevalence of the target disorder or, in the case of prognosis, the prevalence of a positive or negative outcome in a sample population (Chapter 6). The *likelihood ratio* is a summary expression of clinical evidence that predicts either the presence (positive likelihood ratio) or absence (negative likelihood ratio) of the target disorder or outcome; the *posterior odds* represent the *positive predictive value* (calculated from the positive likelihood ratio) or the *negative predictive value* (calculated from the negative likelihood ratio). Multiple likelihood ratios (LR_x) can be combined:

(2) A priori odds × ($LR_1 × LR_2 × LR_3 × \dots LR_x$) = post odds$_x$

As a result, for a given prevalence rate the presence or absence of a series of factors may yield a high negative or positive prediction value. These factors comprise the clinical prediction rule. Before we look at how these rules work, we need to consider the steps that are required to develop a valid clinical prediction rule.

VALIDATION OF A CLINICAL PREDICTION RULE

1. *Was the patient population well defined?* Both diagnostic and prognostic rules apply to specific patient populations. The sample population should be defined by age, sex, and disease process or clinical presentation. For example, a prediction rule for children with suspected bacterial meningitis should come from an observational study of previously healthy children who present acutely with fever and neck stiffness. All of the patients should be assessed for each risk or prognostic factor that will be included in the rule. In ideal cases this data should be collected prospectively, although retrospective data are acceptable if it is complete for the vast majority (>90%) of patients and if it is clear that all of the patients fulfilled well-defined clinical criteria for inclusion. Case-control studies are fraught with covariate bias (unaccounted for risk factors that may be missed and maldistributed because of the retrospective nature of the study) and should be treated as inferior evidence to observational studies.

    The group should also be defined as to source. Because the prevalence rates of diseases and complications may vary with severity and rapidity of the disease process, clinical rules may behave differently when applied to patients who present to emergency rooms, who are hospitalized, who are seen in primary care offices, or who live in diverse geographical locations with varying access to medical care. The source of patients should be similar to the source of patients you plan to evaluate.

2. *Is there a clear definition of the desired clinical or diagnostic outcome?* For a clinical prediction rule to be successful, the "prediction" must be clearly and unequivocally defined. In the case of the Framingham study, the rules predict a clearly identifiable, easily diagnosed, significant cardiovascular event. In other cases, the rule may predict the likelihood of a significant diagnostic test. In general, the rule should predict a clinical or diagnostic outcome that is easily identified and is clearly significant from the patient's point of view. Multiple related outcomes are acceptable as long as they are significant to the patient. The Framingham rules predict not only significant cardiac events but significant cerebrovascular events as well. These rules work because the underlying pathophysiology is similar for both processes.

3. *Is the sample size large enough to identify adequately sized affected and unaffected groups?* To be successful, a sufficiently large group of patients must manifest the clinical or diagnostic outcome of interest. For example, if the outcome of interest has a prevalence rate of 1% in the sample population, several thousand patients will need to be included to generate an affected group

of 20–30 patients. The size of the sample population will vary inversely with the prevalence rate of the outcome of interest.

4. *Was a univariate analysis performed?* To identify quantitative or qualitative differences between those subjects with the target diagnosis or clinical outcome and those without, point-by-point comparisons of individual factors should be performed. These comparisons use traditional statistical techniques to identify differences between the two subject groups. Recently, the technique of *recursive partition analysis* has been used to develop the cutoff points for rule components. This technique randomly samples the population database to generate smaller "sample populations." Each of these sample populations is used to test different cutoff points for each risk factor. The end result is a precise rule that can be tested on the entire sample population. This is a valid way to generate components of the rule.

   Univariate analysis does not distinguish between dependent (outcome) and independent (risk) variables. In the previous chapter, the risk factors for a poor outcome in children with bacterial meningitis included a cerebrospinal fluid white blood cell count less than 1000 cells/mm^3 and age less than 12 months. The cerebrospinal fluid white blood cell count was an outcome (dependent variable) and resulted from the ongoing process of infection. The parameters of a good clinical prediction rule should include only independent variables.

5. *Was a multivariate analysis performed?* A multivariate analysis is a statistical technique that separates dependent from independent variables. Various techniques exist and may be identified as multiple linear regression analysis, multifactor analysis of variance, multiple factor analysis, or simply regression analysis. The end product of such an analysis is a listing of variables, all of which are statistically different between the target subgroup and the remaining subjects.

6. *Was a clinical rule developed?* Clinical decision rules may take a variety of forms based on the number of independent variables (risk factors), the combined or individual discriminatory power of the risk factors, and the prevalence of the target disorder or clinical outcome in the sample population (see Bayes theorem earlier in this chapter). Sometimes the end result is a clinical scoring system that provides a graded risk of outcomes or probability of diagnosis. In other instances, the rule may consist of multiple components all of which must be met in order to make the prediction. *Negative or low-risk prediction rules* are encountered in cases where the outcome or the target disorder occurs uncommonly or rarely. In these situations, the absence of most or all of the risk factors reduces

the probability of the diagnosis or outcome. The rule may be summarized by its sensitivity, specificity, accuracy [(sensitivity + specificity)/2], negative likelihood ratio, or its negative predictive value (NPV). From a clinical point of view, the NPV is the most important characteristic since (1 − NPV) is the error rate of the rule. For a given prevalence rate, a NPV exceeding 92%–95% is clinically useful.

Positive or calculated risk prediction rules are encountered in cases where the outcome or the target disorder occurs commonly. In these situations, scoring systems may be developed to identify high-risk patients. The Framingham study is an example of a calculated risk rule. For positive predictive rules, the positive predictive value behaves in an identical fashion to the negative predictive values discussed earlier.

7. *Was the clinical rule validated?* Once the clinical rule has been developed, it needs to be validated in a second sample population. In many cases, a second study is performed to validate the rule. As a result, two or more studies addressing a specific clinical prediction rule are often found. *When you search the literature for a rule, read the validation study, since it will confirm whether the rule works!* Sometimes, a second sample population will be included in the original report to validate the rule. In either case, a totally separate population should be used to validate the rule. The use of recursive partition analysis is not acceptable for rule validation, since it does not test the rule across a different population gathered at a different point in time.

FINDING AND USING CLINICAL PREDICTION RULES ABOUT PROGNOSIS

Consider the following case:

A 68-year-old man is admitted to the burn unit of your hospital following a fire in a dwelling. On admission he has 40% burns of his body. He is intubated and his chest X-ray shows diffuse changes consistent with inhalation injury. What is the likelihood that this patient will survive his injuries?

Finding the Evidence

For this case, the PubMed clinical queries search engine was used. The radio buttons for clinical prediction rules and narrow search were checked. The search terms "burns" and "outcome" were entered. The search yielded 32 citations; the first citation appeared to address the question.

Table 8-1. Risk Factors and Mortality Risk Scoring for Burn Patients

	SCORE				
Risk Factor	*0*	*1*	*2*	*3*	*4*
Age (y)	<50	50–64	65–79	>80	
Burned Surface Area (%)	<20	20–39	40–59	60–79	>80
Inhalation Injury	No			Yes	

Source. Reprinted with permission from the Belgian Outcome in Burn Injury Study Group. Development and validation of a model for prediction of mortality in patients with acute burn injury. *Br J Surg* 2009; 96:111.

Table 8-2. Score–Risk Table for Burn Patients

	SCORE										
	0	*1*	*2*	*3*	*4*	*5*	*6*	*7*	*8*	*9*	*10*
Predicted mortality (%)	0.1	1.5	5	10	20	30	50	75	85	95	99

Source. Reprinted with permission from the Belgian Outcome in Burn Injury Study Group. Development and validation of a model for prediction of mortality in patients with acute burn injury. *Br J Surg* 2009; 96:111.

Evaluating the Evidence

The Belgian Outcome in Burn Injury Study Group. Development and validation of a model for prediction of mortality in patients with acute burn injury. *Br J Surg* 2009; 96:111. This study evaluated all of the burned patients admitted to hospitals in Belgium between 1999 and 2004. The model was developed (derived) using 5246 patients admitted between 1999 and 2003; the model was validated using patients admitted during 2004 (981). In the derivation cohort, 242 patients died (4.6%). The univariate and multivariate analyses identified age, percent burned surface area, and the presence of inhalation injury as the independent variables for death. The resultant model uses a scoring system based on age, percent burns, and inhalation injury to predict risk of death (Table 8-1). When validated, the receiver–operator curve for the model produced an area under the curve (AUC) of .94. From our past discussion, you may remember that the AUC provides a proxy for the probability that the test will separate positives from negatives. In this case, the AUC suggests that the model is robust.

The independent variables (risk factors) are age, burned surface area, and presence of an inhalation injury. Our patient is 68 years old (2 points), has a burned surface area of 40% (2 points), and has inhalation injury (3 points) for a total of 7 points. The risk is calculated from Table 8-2. Our patient has an *average* predicted mortality rate of 75%.

FINDING AND USING CLINICAL PREDICTION
RULES ABOUT DIAGNOSIS

Consider the following case:

> A 22-year-old man is brought to the emergency room following
> an automobile accident. His past medical history is unremarkable.
> An hour ago, he rear-ended a bus at a traffic light. He said that he
> skidded on the highway and hit the bus at less than 10 miles per
> hour. He did not lose consciousness. He had a glass of wine with
> dinner 2 hours ago (blood alcohol is .02 µg/dl, safe for driving in
> his state is <.08 µg/dl). He has no other injuries. On examination
> he is in a neck collar, provide by the emergency medical techni-
> cians who brought him in. He has no neck pain or other injuries.
> His neurological examination is normal. Does he need an imaging
> study of his neck prior to removal of the protective collar?

Finding the Evidence

For this case, the PubMed clinical queries search engine was used.
The radio buttons for clinical prediction rules and narrow search were
checked. The search terms (C-spine OR "cervical spine") injury, trauma,
and imaging were used; 16 citations were returned. The first appeared to
address the issue.

Evaluating the Evidence

Steill IG, Clement CM, McKnight RD, et al. The Canadian C-spine rule
versus the NEXUS low-risk criteria in patients with trauma. *N Engl J Med*
2003; 349:2510. This study validated two established rules for "clear-
ing" neck injuries without radiographic examination in injured patients:
The Canadian C-Spine rule and the NEXUS low-risk criteria. This study
enrolled 8283 patients in nine Canadian referral centers with head or
neck trauma, visible injuries above the clavicles, no ambulation, history
of a dangerous mechanism of injury, normal vital signs and level of consciousness, and injury within 48 hours of evaluation. Two percent (169
patients) had a significant C-spine injury; the huge number of patients
enrolled in this study was required given the low prevalence rate. All of
the patients were scored according to both the Canadian C-spine rule
(age > 65, paresthesias in the extremities, low-risk mechanisms that permit assessment of range of motion of neck, and active rotation of the neck
45 degrees left and right), and the NEXUS criteria (no midline C-spine
tenderness, no evidence of intoxication or altered mental status, no focal
neurological deficit, and no painful distracting injuries). The performance
of each test is shown in Table 8-3. The Canadian C-spine rule appears to
be more robust and is intrinsically a better rule given the huge difference
in –LR. This translates into a much higher NPV. Since the number of

Table 8-3.   Test Characteristics of the Canadian C-Spine Rule and the NEXUS Criteria for the Prediction of Neck Injuries in Trauma Patients

	Canadian C-Spine Rule	*NEXUS Criteria*
Sensitivity	99.4	90.7
Specificity	45.1	36.8
+ LR	1.81	1.44
– LR	75.17	3.96
PPV	3.56%	2.85%
NPV	98.66%	79.49%

Source. Reprinted with permission from Steill IG, et al. The Canadian C-spine rule versus the NEXUS low-risk criteria in patients with trauma. *N Engl J Med* 349(26):2510–2518. Copyright © 2003 Massachusetts Medical Society. All rights reserved.

patients in this study is so large, the calculated NPV approaches the 95% lower confidence limit for this test, so we can conclude that 95% of the data supports an NPV of 98.7% or greater. The real question is whether the physician wants to use this rule and forgo neck imaging in these patients and accept at most a 1.3% error risk or simply image all patients who present with a dangerous mechanism of injury.

9

ANSWERING A QUESTION ABOUT ETIOLOGY OR DIFFERENTIAL DIAGNOSIS

Identifying the cause of a patient's symptoms is the most important task in clinical medicine. In some cases the cause of the patient's illness is obvious. In other cases, a number of entities may be implicated and a differential diagnosis needs to be developed. Developing a complete differential diagnosis or listing of possible etiologies is difficult. From the patient's point of view, it needs to be complete in order to identify the underlying cause of symptoms as quickly as possible. From the clinician's point of view, the traditional method of generating a differential diagnosis requires an encyclopedic knowledge of disorders, including unusual clinical presentations and epidemiology. In this section, we will discuss the use of translational research in developing a differential diagnosis.

DEVELOPING A DIAGNOSTIC PARADIGM AND FINDING THE EVIDENCE

The starting point for differential diagnosis is the generation of the diagnostic paradigm. Diagnostic paradigms need to be as specific and as precise as possible. Many experts suggest that diagnostic paradigms should include as many contrasting terms as possible. Consider the following example:

> A 46-year-old man presents to the clinic with a 4-day history of rash and fever. He was in his usual state of health until 4 days ago when he developed a low-grade, tactile fever. Three days ago he

began to develop a rash on his arms and trunk. Since then the rash has progressed. The rash is pruritic and he noticed some scaling today. He has no drug allergies and his past medical history is unremarkable. His physical examination is remarkable for a temperature of 38.2°C, bilateral cervical, non-tender lymphadenopathy, and a generalized rash. The rash is flat, confluent, erythematous, blanches, and looks like sunburn. You recall that this type of rash is often referred to as erythroderma. What is the clinical diagnostic paradigm in this case?

To begin, this is an adult, not an infant, child, or adolescent. This is important because it is reasonable to expect that the differential diagnosis will differ among these populations. Next, we need to consider the timing of the onset of the illness: acute (days), subacute (weeks), or chronic (months). Third, we need to identify any underlying diseases, significant past medical history, medications, or allergies. Finally, we need to identify all of the signs and symptoms. In this case, he has fever, rash, and lymphadenopathy. Therefore, as a first pass we can generate the following diagnostic paradigm:

> What is the differential diagnosis of the acute onset of rash, fever, and lymphadenopathy in a previously healthy adult male?

To test this paradigm, make a list of all of the conditions that you can think of that might present this way. How big is your list? Now, go to the clinical queries section of the PubMed page. In the clinical study categories section enter the search terms fever, rash, lymphadenopathy, and adult, click the radio buttons for etiology and broad, sensitive search and perform the search. How many citations did you find? How relevant are these articles to your patient? Now try the same search using the narrow, specific search button instead of the broad, sensitive button. Fewer articles appear. Are any of them relevant to the patient?

It appears that this paradigm is too broad. How can we improve it? A successful clinical paradigm needs to be as specific as possible. Clearly many entities are associated with rash, fever, and lymphadenopathy. We cannot be more specific about the fever or the lymphadenopathy. However, the rash can be described in more specific terms. So let's modify the paradigm to read:

> What is the differential diagnosis of the acute onset of erythroderma, fever, and lymphadenopathy in a healthy adult male?

Now try the clinical query on PubMed using a broad, sensitive search. What did you find? Did you find the following article: Erythroderma: a clinical study of 97 cases, *BMC Dermatol* 2005; 5:5? Print a copy of the article for use in the next section.

VALIDATING THE EVIDENCE

To answer a question regarding etiology or differential diagnosis, the study should answer the following questions:

1. *Is the patient population similar to the patient in question?* The subjects of the study should be clearly described with regard to clinical symptoms and demographics. The clinical symptomatology should be specific. In the study found in the example, all of the subjects presented with erythroderma. The patients included males and females and the average age was 46 years. Since the patient described here meets these criteria, this is an appropriate article. If this had been a study of children, the elderly, or only women, it would not have been valid for the patient in question. A similar problem arises for a study population limited by elements of history (e.g., only patients with documented drug allergies are included) or physical examination (e.g., only patients with accompanying alopecia).

2. *Is the study large enough to provide a complete differential diagnosis?* These studies are of cross-sectional design. No comparison groups are included. Because the studies may be retrospective it should be possible to include a large number of patients. The number of subjects should be driven by the complexity of the differential diagnosis. Symptom complexes with only a limited number of possibilities can be the subjects of much smaller studies than symptom complexes with many more possibilities. In some cases, a search for a specific symptom complex may only yield case reports of specific entities.

3. *Is the diagnostic evaluation described complete and uniformly performed?* A valid study will describe, in detail, specific elements of the medical history, physical findings, and diagnostic evaluation performed on each patient. In the best studies, the diagnostic protocol will be determined at the onset of the study and patients will be collected prospectively. For unusual or relatively rare diagnoses, the diagnostic protocol will be determined prior to the retrospective identification of patients with the symptom complex of interest. In these cases, missing data should be detailed in the Results section. In our example, if a skin biopsy is part of the diagnostic protocol, the authors should note not only how many skin biopsies were diagnostic but what percent of the sample population underwent the procedure.

4. *Is the constellation of clinical signs and symptoms defined for the sample population?* It is not surprising that patients with an illness characterized by a prominent sign or symptom also have other signs and symptoms. In a study of differential diagnosis, these other findings and the incidence of each should be

included. In our example of erythroderma, 94% of the patients
had pruritis, 33.6% were febrile, and 21.3% had lymphadenopathy. Associated laboratory data should also be detailed. If
possible, the association of other findings with each diagnostic
possibility should also be detailed.

5. *Are all of the patients accounted for diagnostically?* At the end of
the study a compilation of etiologies and frequencies is required
in order for the study to be of use. Moreover, diagnoses should
be by disease entity; identification by class of disease only, for
example, drug reaction, malignancy, or autoimmune disorder,
is of much less use. In the example, diagnoses are listed both by
category (previous dermatoses [59.8%], malignancies [11.3%],
and drug reactions [21.6%]) as well as entity (psoriasis [27.8%],
atopic dermatitis [13.4%], etc.). Note that the authors included a
category for idiopathic or undetermined etiology (7.2%) to complete the accounting of all of the patients. One of the distinct
advantages of evidence-based differential diagnosis is an estimate of the percentage of patients who will remain undiagnosed
despite a rigorous workup (apologies to Dr. House).

Individual case reports do not provide enough depth to draw conclusions regarding the relative frequencies of different disorders, nor do they
provide sufficient information to conclude how many patients will remain
undiagnosed. Nevertheless, in some cases, this is the best evidence available and you may have to develop a diagnostic list from a number of case
reports.

10

USING MEDICAL EVIDENCE TO ANSWER A QUESTION REGARDING CLINICAL PRESENTATION

Dr. Carl Gartner was the chief resident of pediatrics at Children's Hospital of Pittsburgh during my senior year of medical school. While rotating as a subintern on one of the inpatient units, we were confronted by a patient with an unusual medical history. Many of the features of the child's illness were consistent with an acute viral infection, an illness that was common in Pittsburgh during the fall. However, several features of the illness did not appear to fit. Carl's approach: "Common diseases present commonly and common diseases present uncommonly." He imparted that wisdom many years ago, but it is still true today.

Many times on rounds, a student or resident will be stymied by the diagnosis for a particular patient. Most of the clinical features fit a single entity, but one or two symptoms are either lacking from the classic description of the disease or seem to be part of some other disease. At this point, most students want to add a second illness to the patient's woes. The Franciscan friar William of Ockham was an English logician who lived in the fourteenth century. His famous principle *entia non sunt multiplicanda praeter necessitatem* translates from Latin as "entities must not be multiplied beyond necessity" and is widely known as Occam's razor. When applied to diagnostic medicine, this rule means that as few entities as possible should be implicated as explanations for a given patient's symptoms (again with apologies to Dr. House). Occam's razor and Dr. Gartner's words of wisdom have always been guiding principles for me when I have been confronted with a diagnostic dilemma.

The previous chapter described a method for using translational research to develop a differential diagnosis. The case example was that of a 46-year-old man who presented with the acute onset of erythroderma, fever, and lymphadenopathy. Evidence from an article in *BMC Dermatology* identified dermatoses and drug reactions as the most common causes. Let's add some additional history and clinical data:

> After talking with the man's wife we discover that he has had a 2-year history of clinically significant trigeminal neuralgia. Contact with his primary care physician reveals that he has been receiving carbamazepine for the past 18 months for this disorder. His admission laboratory data reveal: ALT – 330 u/L (<40 u/L); AST 400 u/L (<40 U/L) and GGTP – 1000 u/L (<100 u/L).

The evidence that we initially found identified carbamazepine as the most common drug associated with fever and erythroderma in adults. So far so good, but what about the elevated liver enzymes? Does this patient have viral hepatitis as well? Could all of his symptoms be caused by viral hepatitis? Does he have an unusual malignancy? How can we figure this out?

At this point, some clinicians would embark on an in-depth diagnostic evaluation that may include a liver biopsy to determine whether the patient has evidence of a viral infection or a malignancy. Dr. Gartner would say "common diseases present uncommonly." Reviewing the list of diagnostic entities associated with the acute onset of fever and erythroderma, you could easily say that none of these disorders are common. In general, that is true but in the universe of this clinical paradigm, primary skin disorders and drug reactions are common diseases. Additionally, carbamazepine is the most commonly implicated drug. Turning to PubMed we enter the term "carbamazepine" and receive a prompt "carbamazepine induced." We select the prompt and add the term "erythroderma." The search yields 14 citations; the first is Ganeva M, et al. Carbamazepine-induced drug reaction with eosinophilia and systemic symptoms (DRESS) syndrome: report of four cases and brief review. *Int J Dermatol* 2008; 47:853. This article describes four patients and reviews several articles on DRESS syndrome. Two of the patients identified in the paper had elevated liver enzymes. A table in the article suggests that up to 60% of patients with DRESS syndrome may have hepatitis. Applying Occam's razor, carbamazepine toxicity appears to be the most likely diagnosis.

In this example, a very small case series provided the evidence needed. In some instances, a single case may be all of the evidence that is available as evidence. What criteria then are needed to validate evidence addressing an issue of clinical presentation?

1. *Was the clinical diagnosis established?* Regardless of the number of patients included in the report, the diagnosis needs to be established rigorously. In the example given, all of the patients

described were receiving carbamazepine, had clinical signs and symptoms previously described with the drug, and responded clinically to removal of the drug. In other cases, definitive diagnostic tests may be needed.

2. *Is my patient like the patients studied?* In this study, all of the patients had erythroderma and fever, similar to the patient at hand. If our patient had lacked the rash, for example, it is not clear that he would have fit the study series. Patient characteristics need to match to ensure that the data from the clinical series are applicable to the patient in question.

3. *Is enough detail provided to determine if the association is supported?* In this case, the values for the liver enzymes were reported. Suppose the authors had simply noted that liver enzymes were "elevated"? Which values were elevated? If GGTP was elevated in our patient but not in those reported in the literature, then the data may support the finding of "hepatitis" in our patient. Degrees of elevation are also important. If the patients in the literature had AST and ALT values in the 150–300 u/L range and our patient's values were in the 3000 u/L range, the literature may not be supportive.

4. *Were other causes of the association excluded?* Even though we all subscribe to Occam's razor, patients do have underlying diseases This is a particular problem when drugs are implicated as the cause of a clinical syndrome. In this case, we can feel comfortable that trigeminal neuralgia is not associated with the constellation of symptoms that comprise the current illness.

Consider the following case:

A 25-year-old man presents to your office to address his complaint of persistent dysuria. He was well until 2 months ago when he noted a tick on his leg while camping in Connecticut. He removed the tick without difficulty and had no rash at the site of the bite. Over the next 2 weeks, he developed a low-grade fever (less than 38.5°C), diffuse back pain, and dysuria. Four weeks after the bite he was seen by his primary care physician who found no abnormalities on physical examination. Laboratory evaluation at that time was remarkable for 10–15 white blood cells/high-power field in a spun urine, a sterile urine culture, and significant IgG antibody against *Borrelia burgdorferri* along with a positive Western blot to show antibody against specific *Borrelia* outer membrane proteins. He was begun on oral amoxicillin for 3 weeks but the dysuria continued. His primary care physician refers him to you with the request that you consider intravenous ceftriaxone to treat this patient's chronic Lyme disease.

This patient raises an interesting question. Is persistent dysuria with pyuria a part of the clinical spectrum of Lyme disease? If it is then this patient may well be eligible for intravenous antimicrobial therapy for chronic Lyme disease. If not, then you are back to the differential diagnosis of dysuria and pyuria in a young, previously healthy man. As usual, we turn to PubMed to begin our search for the answer. Using the main search engine, the search terms "Lyme disease" and "clinical manifestations" were entered. Sixty-six citations were returned. Using the limits search link, humans and English were entered as filters. The second search yielded 53 citations. One of them seems to address the question: Smith RP, et al. Clinical characteristics and treatment outcome of early Lyme disease in patients with microbiologically confirmed Erythema migrans. *Ann Intern Med* 2002; 136:121. This study looked at a case series of 118 patients aged 17–71 years (mean 51 years) who had a history of erythema migrans, the rash uniquely linked to *Borrelia burgdorferri* infections, and confirmation of infection by either culture or nucleic acid amplification (PCR). In this patient population presenting with acute infection and mostly evaluated within the first week of illness, flu-like symptoms were most common and included fever, myalgia, arthralgia, headache, fatigue, and neck stiffness. In this series of 118 patients, none had dysuria or pyuria.

1. *Was the clinical diagnosis established?* Yes. All of the patients had either culture or PCR evidence of infection. Many studies would have accepted simple antibody testing as was done in our patient.
2. *Is my patient like the patients studied?* Good question. Unlike the patients in the case series, our patient did not have erythema migrans, a sine qua non for Lyme disease. Second, our patient does not have microbiologically confirmed disease, although he does have a compatible exposure history (tick bite) and positive antibody titers 4 weeks after the bite. Finally, the patients in this study were examined early in the course of the disease (median 3 days after the onset of the rash). Our patient was sick for several weeks before he sought out medical attention. Since the catalogue of symptoms reflects the early illness, it is conceivable that dysuria and pyuria may occur later in the course of the disease and were simply missed. Alternatively, if less that 1% of patients with Lyme disease have dysuria and pyuria, it may have been missed in a sample of only 118 patients. These last two points call into question the applicability of this study to the patient in question.
3. *Is enough detail provided to determine whether the association is supported?* This is another good question. If the authors had specifically noted that none of the patients had dysuria or pyuria, the lack of association would be much stronger. The lack of

association is only suggested by the fact that these findings are not included in the list of findings detailed in the article.

4. *Were other causes of the association excluded?* It is hard to apply this question to the situation where the evidence does *not* support the clinical finding. Clearly the implication for our patient is either *(1)* our patient has Lyme disease and the dysuria and pyuria are caused by a second disease *or;* *(2)* our patient never had Lyme disease (suggesting that the antibody titers are a false positive) and that all of his symptoms are caused by some other process.

In either case, the final conclusion from the evidence is that we should pursue other diagnostic possibilities to explain the patient's dysuria and pyuria. This case series, then, was helpful in the assessment of this patient's symptoms. Sometimes continued uncertainty is the best you can find and suggests continued searching is warranted.

11

USING META-ANALYSES TO ANSWER A QUESTION OF DIAGNOSIS AND THERAPY

Frequently, a literature search designed to answer a question will yield multiple studies with similar designs and patient populations. Often, the results of these studies are at odds with each other. How do you know which one to follow? Close examination of each study often reveals several things: *(1)* although the subjects in each study are similar, the number of subjects in each study is small; *(2)* the design of each study is similar; *(3)* the outcome variables for each study are similar but not exact; and *(4)* the results often fail to demonstrate a statistical difference. Wouldn't it be nice if we could combine these smaller studies into a larger one with sufficient power to answer the therapeutic question?

In most cases, published meta-analyses address issues of therapy, although questions of diagnosis can also be addressed in this fashion. A *meta-analysis* is a form of cohort study designed to identify all studies, both published and unpublished, that address the clinical question. The data are extracted from each study, expressed in a uniform and meaningful way, and the results from all of the studies are combined statistically. As with studies addressing issues of diagnosis or therapy, meta-analyses must meet criteria for validity.

1. *Does the study address a well-defined clinical question?* Just as a well-defined question is needed to search the literature, a good meta-analysis should begin with a well-defined question. For example, it is difficult to answer the question, "Should infants with croup receive corticosteroid therapy?" A better question is,

"Compared to placebo, do children less than 3 years of age with croup who receive a single dose of dexamethasone have lower hospital admission rates?"

2. *Was a research protocol defined prior to the initiation of the study?* As with any other cohort study, a valid meta-analysis needs to define its "experimental" protocol prior to the initiation of the study. The protocol needs to define the following: *(1)* the types of subjects to be included (e.g., children <3 years of age); *(2)* any disease states (e.g., the acute onset of inspiratory stridor associated with a febrile upper respiratory tract infection *and* initial presentation to an emergency room); *(3)* the experimental groups (e.g., placebo vs. a single-dose dexamethasone); *(4)* the method of assigning patients to experimental groups; and *(5)* the primary outcomes of interest (hospital admission rate, days in intensive care unit, etc.). Sometimes the investigators run a risk of excluding the majority of studies that address an issue because of the inclusion criteria. As a result, the initial inclusion criteria may be vague. The authors should also describe how each study was reviewed for inclusion. Many large studies will also include criteria to assess the quality of each study.

3. *Was an exhaustive search made to discover all relevant articles?* Because a meta-analysis is a "cohort" study, the investigators need to be scrupulously thorough in their search for both published and unpublished studies. The investigators should detail how the search was performed: What search engine was used? What database(s) were searched? What keywords were used? And what was the yield of the search? The investigators should also review the bibliographies of selected papers to search for additional studies that may have been missed by the computerized search.

   Selection bias is a huge problem. *Publication bias* refers to the observation that studies with positive findings are more likely to be published than those with negative findings. Contacting authors of included studies as well as reviewing the abstracts from pertinent national meetings to search for unpublished studies are often required. Using language as a filter in the search is another source for selection bias. Many high-quality studies are published in languages other than English.

4. *Was there an accounting of all of the articles?* After all of the studies have been identified, each study should be reviewed by several investigators to determine whether all of the inclusion criteria have been met. The investigators should list, by criterion, those studies that have been excluded and should end with the number of studies included for final analysis.

   In addition to this final accounting, many investigators will also assign quality values to each study. For example, in a meta-analysis of placebo versus dexamethasone in croup, studies where the investigators were blinded as to treatment arm will be scored higher than those studies where the investigators were not blirded. The division of the final cohort of studies into subgroups by quality permits sensitivity analysis (see below).

5. *Was a summary table included in the meta-analysis?* A complete meta-analysis should contain a summary table. The table should include all of the pertinent data from each study included in the analysis (number of patients, treatment groups, outcomes, adverse events, etc.). A single outcome (often of the yes/no variety) should be included for each study. Multiple outcomes are acceptable if several analyses are performed, each using a different outcome. Many tables will also include pooled result data (e.g., composite cure rates for treatment groups vs. placebo groups). It should be noted that this data, while nice to see, does *not* constitute a valid analysis.

6. *Was a statistical method used to consolidate the data from all of the studies?* The major assumption that underpins the mathematics of meta-analysis is that all of the studies included in the analysis were drawn from the same population. The Mantel-Haenszel method and the inverse variance method assume that each outcome/exposure pair represents a statistical variation around a "fixed effect." Because of the mathematics involved in a meta-analysis, the results are often expressed as an odds ratio (Chapter 2). Graphical representation shows a consistent location of the central estimate for each study relative to unity and is usually depicted in a *Forest plot*. In Figure 11-1, the odds ratios for curing tinea capitis with terbinafine or griseofulvin are compared. An odds ratio of 1 represents ambivalence.

7. *Was heterogeneity determined and addressed?* The proportion of patients with the desired outcome from each study can be compared by contingency table analysis; this is called *the test for heterogeneity*. If no statistical difference among the proportions is found, the studies are deemed to be homogenous and can be combined. In Figure 11-1, the test for heterogeneity was not statistically significant and the studies were combined using the fixed effects model. In some cases, the central points of each study fail to show a consistent pattern; the test for heterogeneity is often statistically significant in these cases, precluding the use of the Mantel-Haenszel method (fixed effects). A second approach was developed based on the assumption that the results reported by each study represent a "random effect." Using this methodology, heterogeneic studies can be combined. The confidence intervals are wider with this method as compared to the fixed effects method, and there is a major caveat to this approach. When studies appear to be heterogeneic, care must be taken to ensure that major differences really do not exist. In the

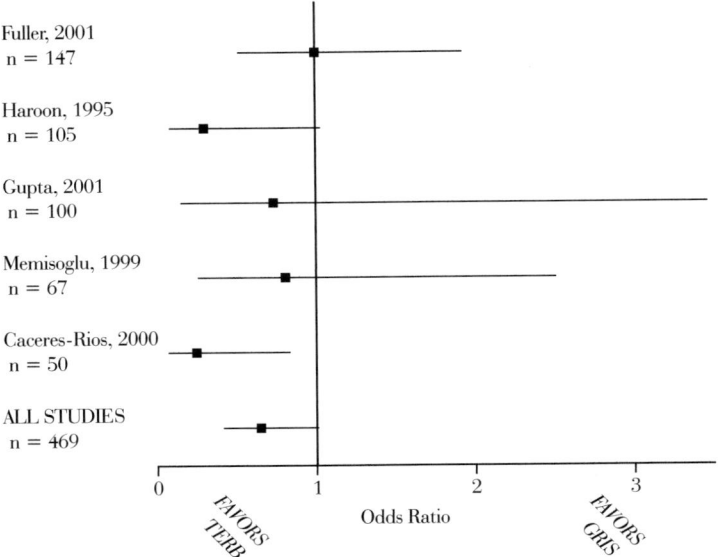

Figure 11-1.   Forest plot of five trials and meta-analysis comparing terbinafine and griseofulvin for the treatment of tinea capitis in children. (Reprinted with permission from Fleece D, Gaughan J, Aronoff, SC. Griseofulvin versus terbinafine in the treatment of tinea capitis: a meta-analysis of randomized, clinical trials. *Pediatrics* 2004; 114:1312–1315.)

study by Fleece et al, where terbinafine and griseofulvin were compared for the treatment of tinea capitis, the original analysis demonstrated marked heterogeneity (Fig. 11-1). On inspection, one study strongly favored the use of griseofulvin over terbinafine while the rest favored terbinafine. In the five studies that comprise the analysis in Figure 11-1, 90% of the isolates from patients were *Trichphyton* species; in the outlier study, 76 % of the isolates were *Microsporum* species. In this case, there was a real reason for the results of one study to differ significantly from the others, and it was valid to exclude the outlier.

8. *Was a sensitivity analysis performed?* Frequently, the cohort of studies identified for the meta-analysis will vary in quality or in fundamental composition. In these cases, it is essential to determine how each individual study affects the outcome of the overall meta-analysis. *Sensitivity analyses* permit these assessments. An example is shown in Figure 11-2. This study examined the ability of serum C-reactive protein concentrations to differentiate bacterial from viral pneumonia in children. The change in overall odds ratio (outcome) when all of the studies were included (row marked none) and with the removal of one

META-ANALYSIS FOLLOWING EXCLUSION OF:	ODDS RATIO (95% CI)	
	RANDOM EFFECT	FIXED EFFECT
NONE	3.54 (1.64–7.66)	Not Applicable
McCarthy, et. al., 1978	2.82 (1.34–5.90)	Not Applicable
Lala, et.al., 2002 (10)	3.50 (1.45–8.41)	Not Applicable
Virkki, et. al., 2002 (11)	4.48 (1.64–12.27)	Not Applicable
Moulin, et. al., 2001 (12)	4.01 (1.32–9.93)	Not Applicable
Heiskanen-Kosma, et. al., 2000 (13)	4.54 (1.94–10.60)	Not Applicable
Korppi, et. al., 1997 (14)	4.09 (1.71–9.75)	Not Applicable
Korppi, et. al.. 1993 (15)	4.01 (1.62–9.94)	Not Applicable
Babu, et. al., 1989 (16)	2.49 (1.42–4.35)	Not Applicable

Figure 11-2. Sensitivity analysis of seven trials evaluating the diagnostic use of C-reactive protein to differentiate bacterial and nonbacterial pneumonia. (Reprinted with permission from Flood RG, Badik J, Aronoff SC. The utility of serum C-reactive protein in differentiating bacterial from non-bacterial pneumonia in children: a meta-analysis of 1230 children. *Pediatr Infect Dis J* 2008; 27:95–99.)

study at a time is shown. In this analysis, the changes in confidence intervals and magnitude of the odds ratio were minimal, demonstrating that no single study was disproportionately influencing the outcome of the meta-analysis. In instances where a single large trial is included in the meta-analysis, the composite outcome may overweight the single trial. Performing an analysis without the large trial will give an indication whether the single large study is affecting the direction of the results. In the example shown in Figure 11-2, the results of the sensitivity analysis strengthen the conclusion that high serum concentrations of C-reactive protein are associated with bacterial pneumonia.

9. *Was publication bias addressed?* One of the major biases encountered in meta-analysis is publication bias. Studies with negative results or with small numbers are less likely to be published than larger studies. One way to graphically determine whether publication bias or selection bias exists is to use a *funnel plot*. This is a plot of some measure of study size (e.g., number of patients in the study) versus the outcome in each study. As seen in Figure 11-3, the spread of central points narrows as the number of patients in the study increases, forming an inverted funnel. Asymmetry in the curve suggests missing studies. Also of interest, the centerline of the funnel approximates the overall odds ratio for the meta-analysis; in the case of Figure 11-3, the

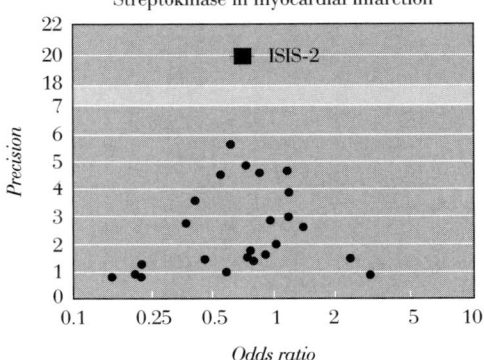

Figure 11-3. Funnel plot of individual small trials and one large trial (ISIS). (Reprinted with permission from Eggar M, et al. Bias in meta-analysis detected by a simple, graphical test. *BMJ* 1997; 315:629–634.)

centerline of the funnel also approximates the odds ratio of a single, huge study (ISIS-2). An alternative method to address publication bias is to calculate the X intercept of the line generated from the plot in Figure 11-3. If the confidence interval for the intercept includes 0, then publication bias is not an issue.

WHERE TO FIND META-ANALYSES

Using PubMed, click on the clinical queries hyperlink. Next, select systematic reviews. Enter your search string on the line provided and launch. A list of appropriate meta-analyses from Medline will be retrieved. Another great source for meta-analyses is the Cochrane Database of Systematic Reviews. This database is searchable via PubMed, but information may only be accessed by subscription or by proxy (OVID, university subscription services, etc).

Now that we have covered the basics, let's look at an example. Consider the following case:

A 4-year-old girl presents to the clinic with the acute onset of urinary frequency and pain on urination. Her mother notes that her urine is particularly foul smelling. A urinalysis is positive for leukocyte esterase, urinary leukocytes, and bacteria. A presumptive diagnosis of acute bacterial cystitis is made. How long should she receive antimicrobial therapy?

Using the systematic review section of the PubMed clinical queries section, the search term "cystitis" is entered. The limits search hyperlink is used to set the limits: human, English, and All Child. Twelve references are returned; one appears to address the issue:

Tran D, Muchant D, Aronoff SC. Short-course versus conventional length antimicrobial therapy for uncomplicated lower urinary tract infections in children: a meta-analysis of 1279 patients. *J Pediatr* 2001;139:93–99.

Although I admit that I shamelessly picked this case since I was an author of the meta-analysis, the impetus for the study was, in fact, the patient described. We picked studies that included patients less than 18 years of age, randomized patients with cystitis to 3 days or less of therapy *or* 5 days or more of therapy and performed quantitative urine cultures prior to therapy and at least 3 days after therapy. Twenty-two studies were found that met these criteria; 17 of these studies used the same drug in the both arms of the study (circles). The Forest plot is shown in Figure 11-4. In this particular case, the data are shown as the difference in percent of patients cured (absolute risk reduction). Because it is expressed as the difference in percentage, it is easily adaptable to the preponderance of evidence method. The random effects method was used for both analyses since heterogeneity was present in both sets of studies. We concluded that the heterogeneity resulted from the large variety of drugs used and the differences in lengths of therapy.

When all of the studies were included, the cure rate with longer courses of therapy exceeded that of the short courses by 6.38% (95% CI: 1.88%–10.89%). When only those studies that matched drugs in both arms of the study were included, the difference was 7.92% (95% CI: 2.09%–13.8%), favoring the longer course of therapy. We can easily apply the method of preponderance of evidence to the data provided. We know that to calculate the 95% confidence intervals 2 standard deviations are added (upper limit) or subtracted (lower limit) from the central tendency value. For all 22 studies, we know that 6.38 − 1.88 = 4.5. Therefore, 2.25 = 1 standard deviation and 1.65 × 2.25 allows us to set the 90% limits. As a result, we can state with 95% certainty that the cure rate with longer therapy is at least 2.7% better than that with shorter therapy, and *on average* 16 patients need to receive longer therapy to prevent one treatment failure than would have occurred with shorter therapy. Overall, longer therapy is better but not that much better. What about the data with matched therapy; after all, comparing the same drugs in short and long courses is probably a better comparison. Using the same method we can conclude with 95% certainty that the cure rate with longer therapy is at least 3.1% better than a shorter course with the same agent; *on average*, 13 patients need to receive the longer course of therapy to prevent one treatment failure that would have occurred with a shorter course of the same agent. These data are a stronger condemnation of short course therapy but many would consider a 3.1% lower limit acceptable, given the convenience of the shorter course and the aggregate cost of the longer course of therapy.

Naturally, we did a sensitivity analysis of our data since there was so much heterogeneity. We found that 5 of the 22 studies compared amoxicillin in both arms and that the difference in cure rates between the two courses was 13% (95% CI: 4%–24%), favoring the longer course. Four of

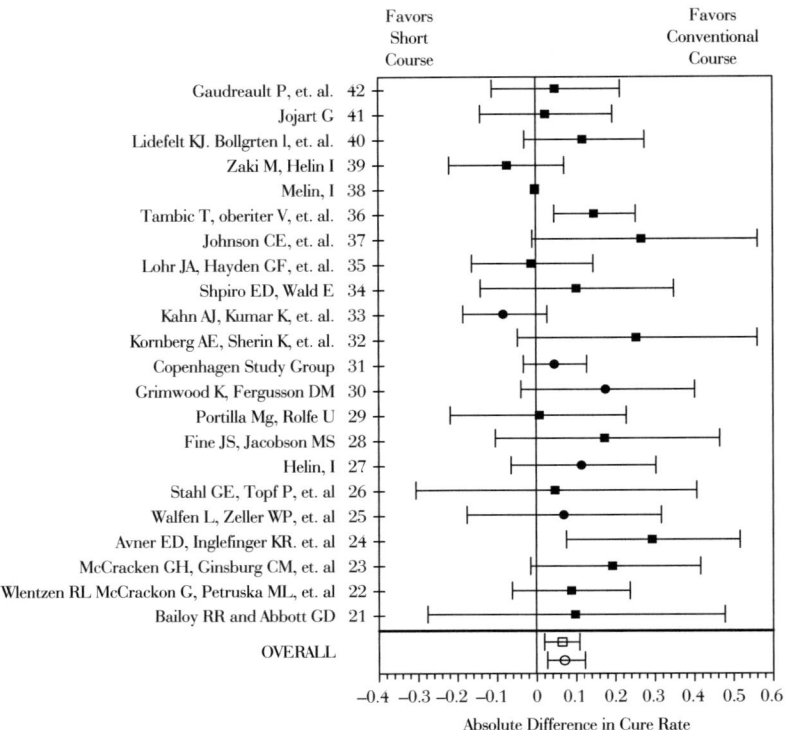

Figure 11-4. Forest plot of individual studies and overall meta-analysis comparing short course and long course antimicrobial therapy for the treatment of uncomplicated urinary tract infections in children. (Reprinted with permission from Tran D, Muchant DG, Aronoff SC. Short-course versus conventional length antimicrobial therapy for uncomplicated lower urinary tract infections in children: a meta-analysis of 1279 patients. *J Pediatr* 2001; 139:93–99.)

these five trials compared a single dose of amoxicillin to 5 or more days of amoxicillin therapy. No significant heterogeneity was found. Therefore, we can state with 95% certainty that the cure rate with the longer course of amoxicillin was at least 5.6% higher than that with short course therapy and, *on average*, eight patients needed to receive the longer course of treatment in order to prevent one treatment failure that would have occurred with a single dose of amoxicillin.

A similar analysis was performed on the six studies that compared short courses and longer courses of trimethoprim-sulfamethoxazole (TMP/SMX); three of these studies used single doses and the remainder used 3 days of therapy. While the overall difference in cure rates favored the longer course of therapy, 6.24% (95% CI: 3.74%–16.2%), we can say with 95% certainty that the longer course is no more than 2% *worse* than short course therapy and no more than 14% *better* than short course therapy. *On average*, 16 patients need to receive the longer course of therapy to prevent 1 treatment failure that would have occurred with the shorter course.

What can we conclude from this study? Using treatment failure as an outcome, short course antimicrobial therapy for uncomplicated cystitis in children is not as good as longer course therapy. In particular, a single dose of amoxicillin is not acceptable therapy, but a short course of TMP/SMX, particularly if you choose 3 days of therapy, is probably adequate therapy. The data on other agents are scant, preventing additional conclusions.

12

ANSWERING A QUESTION REGARDING CAUSATION

In order to establish a causal relationship between two events, a number of criteria need to be met. In the parlance of epidemiology, *exposure* is the term used to describe the causal or inciting event. Administration of a drug, infection with a parasite, and living in an area with high endemic radioactivity are all examples of exposures. *Outcome* is the term used to define the resulting event. Rash, diarrhea, and cancer, respectively, are examples of outcomes as they relate to the exposures cited previously. Typically, the establishment of a causal relationship between an exposure and an outcome is the result of multiple studies. Individual articles may address any of the five criteria required for determining causation; it is difficult for any one study to stand alone given the rigor of the standards that must be met.

1. *Is there a strong exposure–outcome relationship?* The causal relationship between the exposure and the outcome is established by the quality of the study performed. An association can be inferred from the results of a case-control study, a forward in time cohort study (also known as an observational study), or by a randomized clinical trial. The case-control trial is the lowest grade of evidence since it is subject to more bias. In this type of study, subjects are identified by outcome; a control group (without the outcome) is constructed to match the case group, and the frequencies of selected exposures are compared between the groups. Recall and selection bias are major

limitations to this type of study. A cohort study selects patients by exposure (e.g., how close they lived to Chernobyl when it exploded) and then follows them forward in time and measures the frequency of a given outcome in each group (e.g., leukemia). A dose–response curve could be generated from this data by looking at the distance the subject lived from the epicenter of the explosion and comparing outcome rates. Assuming that the dosage of radiation would increase as one moved closer to the epicenter, finding that the incidence of leukemia increased in a similar fashion would provide strong evidence that ionizing radiation can cause leukemia. This type of study is subject to selection and confounding bias. For example, if the poorest families lived closest to the blast and wealthy families lived farther away, economic class may confound the results of the study. Clinical trials, where the investigator randomly assigns subjects to the exposure of interest, provide the best evidence for causation. Not only are these the most difficult and most expensive studies to perform, but in many cases, clinical trials simply cannot be performed (e.g., randomly assigning children to varying doses of ionizing radiation to determine the subsequent risk of leukemia).

2. *Is the association consistent?* To demonstrate causation, the association between exposure and outcome needs to be shown in multiple populations and at multiple times. Reproducibility eliminates investigator error and bias from confounding variables. *Kawasaki disease* is a clinical syndrome of fever, rash, mucositis, conjunctivitis, lymphadenopathy, and swelling of the hands and feet in young children; untreated, approximately 10% of patients develop coronary artery aneurysms. While the cause of this syndrome remains unproven, *Proprionobacterium acne*, toxin-producing *Staphylococcus aureus*, and a host of other factors have been implicated. No single consistent association has been demonstrated to date.

3. *Is the exposure temporally related to the outcome?* If an exposure causes an outcome, then the exposure must precede the outcome in time. Since case-control trials reason backwards in time, reversal of cause and effect becomes a real concern. If the onset of a disease is not well defined or is asymptomatic, the onset of the pathological process may precede exposure. For example, cohort studies of adults with atherosclerosis demonstrated an associated between serum cholesterol levels and the development of symptomatic disease. This led to the recommendation that adults should decrease cholesterol in their diets. Recently, it has been shown that atherosclerotic changes can be found in the vessels of *children* with high serum cholesterol

levels. Therefore, overt cardiovascular disease in adults follows childhood exposure to high levels of cholesterol, suggesting that children should be screened and should undergo dietary therapy. The simple observation that an exposure and an outcome are linked in time is not sufficient evidence to infer causality. As Dr. Edward A. Mortimer, former chairman of epidemiology at Case Western Reserve University pointed out: "Just because it rained last night and you see frogs this morning, don't conclude that it rained frogs." This is the logical fallacy of *post hoc ergo propter hoc* (discussed previously). Those who suggest a causal link between autism and childhood vaccinations have fallen victim to this fallacy.

4. *Is the association between exposure and outcome specific?* To establish causality, an exposure must be both necessary and sufficient to cause the outcome. *Necessary* means that the outcome will not occur in the absence of the exposure. *Sufficient* means that the exposure by itself is all that is required to cause the outcome. In establishing the causes of infectious diseases Koch's postulates, as put forth at the end of the nineteenth century, provided evidence that an infectious agent was necessary and sufficient to cause a disease. Koch required that the infectious agent be recovered from a patient with disease, that the agent be propagated in culture, that the agent be administered to a subject, that the disease occurs in that subject, and that the agent be recovered again from the subject. Modern-day applications of Koch's postulates require that the agent be observed in the patient with disease (by culture or by nucleic acid amplification) and that serologic evidence of infection be found in the vast majority of individuals with the disease.

5. *Is the association between exposure and outcome biologically plausible?* Despite meeting all of the criteria cited earlier, the association between exposure and outcome must make sense biologically. In one large, case-controlled study of children with Kawasaki disease, a history of recent rug shampoo exposure was obtained significantly more often from cases than controls. Subsequent studies examined antibody titers to carpet mites and failed to find a correlate. As such, it is hard to conclude that recent rug shampooing is a cause of Kawasaki disease. Basic science studies may provide a biologic basis for many etiologies. The role of staphylococcal toxin as a cause of Kawasaki disease is supported by the basic science observations that establish this protein as a superantigen, capable of eliciting a broad based inflammatory reaction in the host. Similar data are lacking for *Proprionobacterium*, another etiological candidate for Kawasaki disease.

ESTABLISHING CAUSALITY

Let's look at an example. Cat scratch disease (CSD) was first identified as a distinct clinical entity in 1950. ("Cat Scratch Fever," on the other hand, was a song recorded by Ted Nugent in the 1980s). Suspected to be of infectious origin since its description, it was not until 1983 that small, gram-negative bacilli were seen microscopically in silver-stained lymph nodes from patients with the diagnosis (*Science* 1983; 221:1403). In 1988, a group working at the Armed Forces Institute of Pathology recovered a gram-negative bacterium from the infected lymph nodes of 10 of 19 patients with clinically apparent CSD (*JAMA* 1988; 259:1347). Moreover, 3 of 7 patients with recent onset CSD had significant serum antibody titers to the organism. The organism was subsequently named *Afipia felis* in honor of the institute where it was discovered and the presumed disease that it caused.

Now at this point, many of us would accept *A. felis* as the cause of CSD. The organism was seen in infected tissue, recovered from infected tissue, and elicited an antibody response. In 1992, a group of investigators at the Centers for Disease Control and Prevention who were interested in the cause of bacillary angiomatosis, a disease seen in HIV-infected individuals and caused by *Rochalimaea* (now *Bartonella*) *henselae*, developed a rapid test for measuring antibodies to this organism (*Lancet* 1992; 339:1443). Because of clinical similarities between bacillary angiomatosis and CSD, they looked for antibody to *B. henselae* in sera from 41 patients with CSD and 107 healthy patients with their new test. Eighty-eight percent of the patients with CSD had antibody titers over 1:64, and 94% of the healthy patients had titers under 1:64; moreover, human sera with high antibody titers to *B. henselae* did not react to *A. filis*.

Ok, so which organism causes CSD? An outbreak of CSD in Connecticut supplied part of the answer. In 1991, two children with encephalitis due to CSD were hospitalized in Connecticut (*N Engl J Med* 1993; 329:8). Using standard case definitions and questionnaires, 60 cases of CSD were identified prospectively; 56 of these patients were matched to controls without the disease. The incidence of cat–human interactions was markedly greater among the patients than controls. Eighty-four percent of the CSD patients had serum titers to *B. henselae* exceeding 1:64; only 3.6% of the controls had titers that high. In addition, 81% of serum samples from the patients' cats were seropositive for *B. henselae* as compared with 38% of control cats. Another study, performed at Tripler Army Hospital, looked at seropositivity to *A. felis* and *B. henselae* in 38 patients with clinical CSD (*J Pediatr* 1995; 127:23). All patients had an acute serum titer to *B. henselae* exceeding 1:64; 1 of 48 controls had a positive serum titer of 1:64. Twenty-nine of these CSD patients had serum tested for *A. felis*; none of them were positive. Serological data from cats paralleled the findings in patients. Another study published in 1993 had similar findings.

Although Koch's postulates have never been met for CSD, this body of data supports *B. henselae* rather than *A. filis* as the causative agent of CSD. This organism has been demonstrated repeatedly in the host animals and in patients. It is rarely found in controls. It has not been recovered in culture and reintroduced into a host to produce the disease. Nevertheless, most clinicians regard *B. henselae* as the etiology of CSD. Let's look at a second, more dramatic example. In 1984, the Australian gastroenterologist Barry Marshall identified curved bacilli in mucosal biopsies from 58 of 100 consecutive patients with gastritis, and duodenal and gastric ulcers; gram-negative bacilli were cultured from 11 of these specimens (*Lancet* 1984; 1:1311–1314). Several other reports in both adults and children with gastritis, and gastric or duodenal ulceration confirmed this observation. In 1985, Koch's postulates were fulfilled in dramatic fashion. Dr. Marshall, who was healthy and had no history of gastrointestinal or peptic ulcer disease, underwent gastric endoscopy. The results, not surprisingly, failed to show any evidence of inflammation and no bacteria were cultured from the specimens. One month later, he ingested a live culture of organisms (total dose of approximately 10^9 organisms) recovered from a patient with gastritis. Eight days after ingestion he developed vomiting and became ill. He underwent a second gastroscopic procedure 10 days after ingestion of the culture; mucosal biopsy showed inflammation and culture yielded the same gram-negative organisms. On day 14, treatment was started and the symptoms resolved (*Med J Australia* 1985; 142:436). This remarkable (some would say bizarre) report established *Helicobacter pylori* as the causative agent of chronic gastritis and peptic ulcer disease. Needless to say, this standard for causality is rarely met given the inherent issues with informed consent.

13

CLINICAL GUIDELINES: PREPACKAGED MEDICAL DECISION MAKING

Up to this point, the discussion has focused on how to adapt primary clinical research to medical decision making. The vast majority of primary studies require manipulation in order to use them in this process. One category of evidence that can be used "right out of the box" is clinical guidelines. In general, clinical guidelines may be brief, pertaining to a single element of disease management; or comprehensive, detailing all aspects of a disease from diagnosis to management to follow-up to prevention. Clinical guidelines represent the recommendations of a panel of experts usually selected by an organization of physicians such as the American Academy of Pediatrics, the American College of Cardiology, the Infectious Diseases Society of America, and the American College of Surgeons, to mention just a few. Although these are just "guidelines," you should be aware that in both the clinical and legal worlds, guidelines supported by organizations of this level usually constitute the standard of care. I will provide an example where that may not be the case. In any event, if you are managing a case where appropriate, specific guidelines exist, you should have good evidence to support any action to the contrary.

While the format of clinical guidelines can vary from organization to organization, most contain some fundamental elements. The clinical practice guidelines for the diagnosis and management of intravascular catheter infections (IVC guidelines, for short), prepared by the Infectious Diseases Society of America, is an excellent example of guidelines (*Clin Infect Dis* 2009; 49:1–45).

1. *Who prepared the guidelines?* In most cases, the recommendations contained within a guideline paper represent a consensus of an expert panel. In the case of the IVC guidelines, the panel members represented a variety of other, interested organizations such as the Society for Critical Care Medicine, the American Society of Nephrology, and the European Society of Clinical Microbiology and Infectious Diseases, to name a few. Other guidelines may come from a subgroup within a single organization such as the Committee on Infectious Diseases of the American Academy of Pediatrics. You should be able to convince yourself that the members of the panel have a unique expertise in the topic they are reviewing.

2. *How was the evidence for the guidelines identified?* This section of the guideline is reminiscent of the literature search and protocol development for a meta-analysis. In the case of the IVC guidelines, the database, the search terms, and the dates of search are presented in the paper.

3. *How were the guidelines developed?* The IVC guidelines were developed through a conferencing process. The group defined the questions to be addressed by the guidelines and then tasked individuals or subgroups to address and write individual guidelines. The panel, as a group, reviewed each guideline in draft form. External reviewers were asked to comment on the drafts and to provide comments. When the guidelines were finalized, they were sent to the constituent societies for approval and endorsement. Finally, the completed guidelines went to the parent organization, the Infectious Diseases Society of America (IDSA) for final approval and endorsement. In many cases, guidelines will be supported and endorsed by a variety of organizations. The same guidelines may appear in print in multiple journals, usually the official organs of the endorsing organizations. For example, the most recent guidelines for the prevention of infective endocarditis appeared in *Pediatrics* (the official journal of the American Academy of Pediatrics) and *Circulation* (the official journal of the American Heart Association). This is the only time that multiple publication of the same material is permitted by journal editors.

4. *Was the strength of each recommendation given?* As you look through the guidelines paper from the IDSA, in both the executive summary and the body of the paper each of the 123 recommendations is accompanied by a code. For example, recommendation 11: "Obtain blood samples for blood culture prior to the initiation of antibiotic therapy (A-I)." The code at the end of the recommendation is the strength of the recommendation. For these guidelines, the following codes apply (IDSA and United States Public Health Service USPHS

Grading System as adapted from the Minister of Public Works and Government Services, Canada):

Strength of Evidence

A. Good evidence to support a recommendation for or against use
B. Moderate evidence to support a recommendation for or against use
C. Poor evidence to support a recommendation

Quality of Evidence

  I. Evidence from ≥1 randomized, controlled trial
 II. Evidence from ≥1 well-designed clinical trial without randomization; from a cohort or case-controlled analytic series; from multiple time series (case series); or dramatic results from uncontrolled experiments
III. Evidence from opinions of respected authorities, based on clinical experience, descriptive studies, or reports of expert committees

Recommendation 11 is based on the highest strength and quality of evidence. However, not all guidelines provide the level of evidence that supports the guidelines. The American Academy of Pediatrics, like other medical specialty organizations, frequently issues policy statements on a host of subjects. For example, in October 2009, the Academy issued a policy statement entitled "Guidelines for the Care of Children in the Emergency Department" (*Pediatrics* 2009; 124:1233). A host of guidelines, mostly administrative, were provided addressing the roles of supervisory personnel, requirements for support staff, and requirements for equipment, drills, and transport, just to mention a few. Several other professional organizations endorsed these guidelines as well. An extensive bibliography with citations was provided, but no attempt was made to provide grades of strength for each recommendation.

Let's consider the following case:

An 8-month-old girl presents to the office with 3 days of unexplained fever and fussiness. As part of the evaluation, a urinalysis is obtained and is positive for leukocyte esterase and nitrites. A culture is obtained and the child is started on oral amoxicillin. The mother returns with the infant 2 days later. The child is well and without symptoms. The urine culture was positive for 10^5 CFU/mL of *E. coli* sensitive to amoxicillin. What evaluation of the urinary tract is appropriate at this time?

Using PubMed and the clinical queries tool, the search string "urinary tract infection" is entered. Using the limits hyperlink, the following limits are entered: human, English, All Child, and practice guideline. Twelve citations are returned. The recommendations from the American Academy of Pediatrics are chosen.

The evidence: Practice parameter: the diagnosis, treatment, and evaluation of the initial urinary tract infection in febrile infants and young children. American Academy of Pediatrics. Committee on Quality Improvement. Subcommittee on Urinary Tract Infection. *Pediatrics* 1999; 103:843.

1. *Who prepared the guidelines?* These guidelines were prepared by the committee on Quality Improvement and the Subcommittee on Urinary Tract Infection of the American Academy of Pediatrics. There is no representation or endorsement from any other professional organization. In the world of pediatrics, recommendations from the American Academy of Pediatrics are regarded as gold standards and are acceptable with just the one endorsement.

2. *How was the evidence for the guidelines identified?* Evidence was gathered from the MEDLINE database using a "comprehensive search" strategy and covering the years 1966 to 1996.

3. *How were the guidelines developed?* These guidelines were developed using a standardized decision analysis model with patient risk and cost as outcomes. A threshold approach was used where a given value in the decision model is changed until an alternative strategy is indicated. Based on that value and the remainder of the model, the expert panel examined the data and made recommendations based on consensus. The final product was an algorithm for decision making.

4. *Was the strength of each recommendation given?* Each recommendation was assigned a rating of strong, good, fair, or opinion/consensus by the subcommittee methodologist. This method is not as transparent as the method used by the IDSA in the catheter associated infection guidelines. On the other hand, as we read through the guidelines a detailed discussion of the rationale behind each recommendation is given.

Based on our four-point analysis, we have decided to use these guidelines. Since these guidelines are comprehensive and address almost all aspects of urinary tract infections in young children, we will flip through the pages and try to find the section that addresses postinfection evaluation. Recommendation 11 seems to address this point and reads, in part: "Infants and young children who have the expected response to antimicrobials should have a sonogram and either a voiding cystoureterogram (VCUG) or radionuclide cystography performed at the earliest convenient time (strength of evidence: fair)." Based on these recommendations, we should schedule our patient for a renal ultrasound and a VCUG.

While many consider guidelines to be the final word on clinical decisions, do not assume that guidelines always represent the best evidence available. The pediatric urinary tract infection guidelines were published in 1999 and represent evidence that was available in MEDLINE in 1996, more than 13 years ago. A quick search of MEDLINE from 1996 to present is in order to make sure no new information is available. Using the clinical queries tool, we click *diagnosis* and *narrow search* and enter the search terms "urinary tract infection" and "imaging." Using the limits hyperlink we select the following limits: human, English, all child. The search returns seven citations, including the following: Hoberman A, Charron M, Hickey RW, Baskin M, Kearney DH, Wald ER. Imaging studies after a first febrile urinary tract infection in young children. *N Engl J Med* 2003 Jan 16; 348(3):195–202. Since this study was published in 2003, it was not included in the literature review used to develop the American Academy of Pediatrics guidelines. Applying the rules for the evaluation of a study that addresses the question of diagnosis you find that this is a valid study with the following clinical bottom lines:

1. Twelve percent of 309 children had an abnormality demonstrated by renal ultrasound. Of those children with abnormalities, two cases of hydronephrosis and one case of renal calculi were identified. The remainder of the anatomic abnormalities was inconsequential or would have been identified on fetal ultrasounds obtained routinely during pregnancy.
2. Although 38% of the children had an abnormal VCU, only vesicoureteral reflux was found. At present it is not clear that prophylactic antibiotic therapy for reflux has value.

A basic tenet of medical practice is that the results of a diagnostic test should alter the management of the patient. Since that may not be the case for VCU, we should consider sparing our patient the discomfort and expense of this test. If the results of the fetal ultrasound of our patient are still available, we may be able to avoid the renal ultrasound as well.

The take-home message is simply this. Guidelines endorsed by professional organizations are precisely that: guidelines. Guidelines are not written in stone and are subject to change based on new evidence. While the content of topical guidelines is revisited from time to time, revisions do not necessarily occur in a timely fashion with regard to individual patient care decisions. It remains the practitioner's responsibility as well as the professional and moral obligation to the patient to apply the best standards of care *as available at the time of illness*. Relying exclusively on care guidelines is not always consistent with these responsibilities and obligations. A general search of the literature, not just a search for guidelines, is always required.

14

PUTTING IT ALL TOGETHER

By this time you should be familiar with question formulation, database searching, and validating the types of studies that you will encounter in your day-to-day dealings with patients. You are probably wondering how to put all of this information together so that you can form a conclusion that will affect patient care. The evidence-based medicine community has developed the concept of the Critically Appraised Topic or CAT. A number of websites contain libraries of CATS (http://www.ebmny. org/cats.html and http://www.med.unc.edu/medicine/edursrc/!catlist. htm). There are also a number of ways to construct CATS. Let's look at an example and how the results can be summarized using a simple template. Consider the following case:

> During an outpatient rotation in medicine, you are asked to see a 65-year-old man with a history of diabetes and previous myocardial infarction requiring revascularization. He has been compliant with therapy for his diabetes. On examination, he appears well and his examination is normal except for a blood pressure of 155/96. A review of his chart shows a similar blood pressure value from his last two visits. After discussing the case with your attending, it is clear that your patient is a candidate for two-drug therapy. Although angiotensin-converting enzyme inhibitors (ACEI) or calcium channel blockers (CCB) are often combined with a diuretic, such as hydrochlorthiazide (HCT), given the risk factors in this case, you wonder whether this is optimal therapy.

To begin, we need to define an appropriate clinical question. One question generated by a third-year student when given this case was: "In a patient with a history of myocardial infarction and diabetes mellitus requiring two-drug therapy for hypertension, would a combination of ACEI and CCB be more effective than an ACEI and HCT in reducing subsequent cardiovascular events?" Using the Clinical Queries engine of PubMed with the narrow search radio button clicked, the following search terms were entered: "hypertension," "high risk," "combination therapy," "angiotensin converting enzyme inhibitors." A number of studies were returned, but one seemed particularly useful: Jamerson K, et al. Benazepril plus amlodipine or hydrochlorthiazide for hypertension in high-risk patients. *N Engl J Med* 2008; 359:2417. Portions of this article were discussed in Chapter 2.

Using the techniques described in Chapter 2, the following information can be gleaned from the article:

1. As noted in Chapter 2, the last paragraph of the introduction contains the statement "The ACCOMPLISH study was a multicenter, double-blind, clinical trial that compared the rates of morbidity and mortality from cardiovascular causes when two different combination therapies were used as the initial trial intervention in patents with hypertension who were at high risk for a cardiovascular event." Since our patient has two conditions which place him at high risk (diabetes and previous myocardial infarction), the results of this study may be applicable to his care. In the next section of the paper, prior coronary events and diabetes are listed as high risk factors for hypertensive patients included in the study.

2. Patients were recruited from 548 different centers, mostly in Scandinavia. The study was powered to detect a 15% reduction in outcome rate with a power of 90%.

3. Five thousand seven hundred forty four (5744) patients received benazepril (ACEI) + amlodipine (CCB) daily, and 5762 received benazepril (ACEI) + hyrdochlorthiazide (HCT) daily. Only nine patients dropped out.

4. Patients were *randomized*, and investigators and patients were *blinded* as to assignment.

5. *The primary outcome* was the time to the first cardiovascular event defined as myocardial infarction, stroke, hospitalization for unstable angina, coronary revascularization, or sudden cardiac arrest. Events could be fatal or nonfatal. The mean duration of treatment administration was 30 months.

   a. The primary outcome rate in the ACEI + CCB group was 9.6% (552/5744) and in the ACEI + HCT group was 11.8% (679/5762). The rate ratio was 1.22 (90% CI: 1.13–1.33) and the absolute risk reduction was .02 (number needed to treat (NNT) = 46).

b. The death rate over the observed period of time was 4.1%
(236/5744) in the ACEI + CCB group and was 4.5%
(262/5762) in the ACEI + HCT group. The rate ratio was
1.10 (90% CI: .96–1.26), and the absolute risk reduction was
.0044 (NNT = 228).

The CAT template is a wonderful way to summarize and analyze this
study. The CAT for this study is shown as CAT 1. The first section is a
description of the patient. This part should be short and should contain
a statement of the patient's problem and all of the salient history. In this
example, the problem is the patient's hypertension, and the most important historical facts are the two risk factors for cardiovascular complications of high blood pressure. The next section is a statement of the clinical
question raised by the patient. In this case, the question is one of management and it follows the PICO format: Patient, Intervention, Comparison,
and Outcome. The format can be adjusted for different types of questions
as we will see later.

CAT 1

Jamerson K, et al. Benazepril plus amlodipine or hydrochlorthiazide for
hypertension in high-risk patients. *N Engl J Med* 2008; 359:2417.

Patient

A 65-year-old male with a history of previous myocardial infarction and
diabetes mellitus presents now with primary hypertension.

Question

In a middle-aged man at high risk for cardiovascular complications of
hypertension, would his risk be lower with an ACEI combined with a
CCB or with HCT?

Search Strategies

Search Engine: PubMed/Clinical queries
Database: Medline
Key Words: Hypertension, high risk, combination therapy, angiotensin
converting enzyme inhibitors
Filters: Therapy, narrow search, English, middle aged

Study Summary

Study Type: Clinical trial
Study Population: Middle-aged individuals with hypertension and risk
factors for cardiovascular events.
Intervention: ACEI + CCB

Comparison: ACEI + CCB

Outcome Measures: Primary outcome was the total number of fatal and nonfatal cardiovascular events at an average treatment time of 30 months.

Clinical Bottom Lines

1. The event rate for those receiving ACEI + CBB was 9.6% and for those receiving ACEI + HCT was 11.8%. Likelihood ratio = 1.22 (90% CI: 1.13 –1.33). The absolute risk reduction was .02 (NNT = 46).

2. The mortality rate for those receiving ACEI + CCB was 4.1% and for those receiving ACEI + HCT was 4.5%. Likelihood ratio = 1.10 (90% CI: .96 – 1.26). The absolute risk reduction was .0044 (NNT = 228).

Validity Criteria

1. *Were the subjects well defined at the time of enrollment?*   Yes.
2. *Was there an appropriate control group?*   Yes.
3. *Were patients effectively randomized to treatment or control?*   Yes.
4. *Was a significant outcome selected?*   Yes.
5. *Were all patients accounted for at the conclusion of the study?*   Yes.
6. *Was an intent to treat analysis performed?*   No, but there were only nine dropouts out of a sample population of more than 11,000 patients.
7. *Was the power of the study determined?*   Yes, .90 to detect a 15% reduction in rate (rate of 9.78% or less in ACEI + CCB group to be valid).
8. *Were the investigators and subjects blinded as to group assignment?*   Yes.

The search strategy should contain enough information so that the search can be duplicated. The search engine, database, search strings, and filters should be identified. The study summary begins with the identification of study type. In Chapter 3, the different types of study designs were discussed. This study was a clinical trial. The remainder of the study summary also follows the PICO format. Always identify the primary outcome since clinical trials are powered by the primary outcome. Additional outcomes often require an analysis of a subset of patients, reducing the number of subjects and, as a consequence, the power of the study. Alternatively, the prevalence rate of secondary outcomes may be less than that of the primary outcome, again reducing the power of the subanalysis. In either case, secondary outcomes are less important analytically and often fall to the level of passing interest. The clinical bottom lines should relate directly to the primary outcome; clinically significant secondary outcomes may also be included. As noted earlier, likelihood ratios (rate ratios) are the preferred outcome measurement. The mean value with its 90% confidence intervals should be given for the primary outcome. Since this is a clinical trial, the absolute rate reduction and the number needed to treat are also given for the primary outcome. In the example, mortality was a secondary outcome and was included since it is an important outcome. Finally, the study needs to be validated. The validation criteria for the different types of clinical questions have been outlined in each of the preceding chapters. The easiest way to validate a study is to answer each of those questions as shown in the CAT.

Using the Evidence

Now that the pertinent information from the study is in a nice, neat package, a conclusion must be drawn and a medical decision must be made and explained to the patient.

Drawing a Conclusion

In the world of medical decision making, the final conclusion of a critically appraised topic is a single, declarative statement that encompasses the applicability, validity of design, integrity of design, and results. The CAT on hypertension will be used to illustrate these points.

1. *Do the results of this study apply to my patient?* The patient is a middle-aged male with new-onset hypertension and two risk factors for significant cardiovascular complications. The description of the study population includes patients with risk factors like the patient in question. In this case, possible geographic differences (our patient is in the United States and most of the study patients were in Scandinavia) are trivial. In cases where significant differences exist between the patient in question and the study population, a decision must be made as to the applicability of the study. For example, if all of the patients in the study were middle-aged women from Scandinavia, the results of the study may not be readily applicable to the index patient. Conversely, if all of the patients in the study had chronic renal failure and the patient in question did not, then we could conclude that the study has no applicability and no further analysis would be needed. Not surprisingly, some cases will be clear cut and others will not. Moreover, cases will occur where the only evidence that exists is in a study population that only vaguely resembles the index patient.

2. *Is the design of the study valid for the clinical question raised?* As discussed in Chapter 3, a number of different study designs exist. In the example, the clinical question is one of therapy or treatment. The optimum study design is the clinical trial. To qualify as a clinical trial, a patient population must be identified by a

uniform set of criteria (in this case, hypertensive patients with risk factors), gathered together at the beginning of the study (forward in time), and entered into an a priori study protocol assigned to separate groups using a scheme devised by the investigator. Alternative study designs, such as a forward in time observational study where patients are assigned to groups by treating physicians or a backward in time case-control study, suffer from selection bias and provide weak and possibly unreliable results. For questions of therapy, these types of alternatively designed studies support clinical trials when the results are similar; when the results are disparate, clinical trials trump studies of other designs. Unfortunately, there are cases where alternatively designed studies may be the only evidence available. In our example, the study design was a clinical trial and it met the criteria for validity of design.

3. *Is the design of the study internally valid?* The last section of the CAT lists the eight criteria for a high-quality clinical trial. The example is a high-quality study since all eight of the criteria were met. Whether the results of a "less than perfect" study should be accepted and applied to patient care is a judgment that falls to the care provider. In some cases, a flawed study is the best evidence available.

4. *What do the results of the study show?* Since this study clearly is applicable to our patient and is both externally and internally valid, we can now turn our attention to the results. Looking at the primary outcome, ACEI + CCB was statistically more effective than ACEI + HCT, but the clinical significance depends on what threshold is chosen. As noted in Chapter 5, clinical significance requires 84%–95% confidence in an outcome difference of at least 15%. From the data generated by the study, patients receiving ACEI + HCT are 22% more likely to suffer a cardiovascular event, *on average*, than patients receiving ACEI + CCB. So far so good. By the rule of preponderance of evidence, we can say with 95% certainty that the increased risk for the ACEI + HCT group is at least 13%, barely missing clinical significance. Accepting a lower degree of certainty, we can say with 84% certainty that the increased risk for the ACEI + HCT group is at least 16%, surpassing the 15% threshold. Finally, a whopping 46 patients *on average* need to receive ACEI + CCB in order to avoid one cardiovascular event that would have occurred if ACEI + HCT were used instead.

Fatality was a secondary outcome in this study but clearly an important one. We can say with 95% certainty that ACEI + CCB was no more than 4% worse than the HCT combination. *On average*, 228 patients needed to receive ACEI + CCB to prevent one death that would have occurred with the use of ACEI + HCT.

So what conclusions can be drawn from this study? To say that ACEI + CCB is at least as good as ACEI + HCT in this patient population is an understatement and is overly conservative. To say that ACEI + CCB is superior to ACEI HCT is, to me, an overstatement given that the 84% threshold barely achieves clinical significance, that the midpoint value does not exceed 25%, and that the number needed to treat is huge at 46. Thus, a good conclusion for this study would be: *High-risk hypertensive patients who receive ACEI + CCB experience a marginally lower rate of fatal and nonfatal cardiovascular events than those who receive ACEI + HCT.*

Decision Making and Patient Discussion

The final step in medical decision making is, obviously, making the decision. Once a course of action has been determined, it must be explained to the patient. In this case, it is reasonable to begin therapy with two drugs, an ACE inhibitor and a calcium channel blocker. How would you explain this to the patient? I would begin by telling the patient that he has high blood pressure. Untreated, the hypertension, along with his diabetes and previous heart attack, places him at a great risk for another heart attack. We can reduce that risk significantly by using two agents to control his blood pressure. I would go on to say that studies show that one combination of agents, ACE inhibitors and calcium channel blockers, reduces the risk a tiny bit more than other combinations in large numbers of patients. Finally, I would tell him that I would like to start these medications today and see him back soon to make sure that his blood pressure is coming down.

Let's look at an example that addresses a question of diagnosis. As part of the Temple Medical Decision Making Curriculum, students are presented with a case and asked to generate a CAT during the didactic portion of the course. After completion of the didactic material, each student is expected to identify clinical issues from patients seen during the clerkship and to generate appropriate CATs. CAT 2 was generated independently by a third-year medical student rotating on Family Medicine as part of the curriculum in "Medical Decision Making":

CAT 2

Ahmad CS, McCarthy M, Gomez J, Shubin B. The moving patellar apprehension test for lateral patellar instability. *Am J Sports Med* 2009; 37:4.

Patient

A 16-year-old male presents with a complaint of knee instability and pain following a tackle and a fall during a neighborhood football game today. On physical examination, he had a positive patellar instability test.

Question

What is the positive predictive value of the patellar instability test?

Search Strategies

Search Engine: PubMed
Database: Medline
Key Words: Patellar instability test, cohort study
Filters: None

Study Summary

Study Type: Retrospective cohort
Study Population: 51 patients who underwent knee surgery for suspected patellar instability
Intervention: Results of patellar instability test
Comparison: Dislocation of patella under anesthesia at surgery
Outcome Measures: Not applicable

Clinical Bottom Lines

1. The prevalence of patellar dislocation by examination under anesthesia was 49% (25/51). One hundred percent of the patients with patellar dislocation had a positive instability test (Sensitivity = 100%); 23 of 26 patients without patellar dislocation had a negative test (Specificity = 88.4%).
2. The positive likelihood ratio for the patellar instability test was 8.33 and the positive predictive value was .89. The 90% lower confidence limit was .82.
3. The negative likelihood ratio for the patellar instability test was 88 (estimate) and the negative predictive value was .99. The 90% lower confidence limit was .97.

Validity Criteria

1. *Has the diagnostic test been evaluated in an appropriate patient sample?*   Yes, the patient sample is appropriate since the test would generally only be done on people with complaints of anterior knee pain and instability.
2. *Has each patient in the cohort been evaluated by both the gold standard test and the test in question?*   Yes.
3. *Does the cohort include patients with diseases that may be confused with the target disorder?*   Yes.
4. *Have the reproducibility of the test results and its interobservational variation been determined?*   No, since the test was only performed by one person.
5. *Have all of the terms used in the study been defined?*   Yes.
6. *If the test is part of a series of tests, has its contribution to the series been determined?*   No.

Submitted by Brian Canfield

Do the results of this study apply to the index patient? Probably yes since the patient population consisted of individuals with anterior knee pain and instability. The qualification of this answer centers on the fact that all of the subjects in the study underwent attempted dislocation of the knee under anesthesia at the time of surgery. An issue of selection bias must be raised, since it is not clear what the indication was for surgery in the sample population. If, for example, it was the practice of the investigators to operate on all patients with suspected patellar dislocation based on the results of the patellar instability test, then these results would apply to the index patient. If, however, other indications for surgery were used (e.g., a displaced femur fracture accompanied by a suspected patellar dislocation), then the results may not apply to the patient in question.

Is the design of the study valid for the question raised? Yes, but again a qualification needs to be added. A "retrospective cohort" study suggests that patients were identified, probably from a search of some hospital database, and then data were gleaned from the patients' medical record. This approach creates two potential biases. If the medical record is incomplete or unclear, *recall bias* becomes a problem. The investigators may try to remember what the examination revealed or other pertinent information. *Selection bias* becomes a problem since patients may have been missed in the database search (random bias) or may have been missed because of an alternate diagnosis (systemic bias). Ideally, all patients over a given period of time who present with anterior knee pain and joint instability should have been included in the study. While these problems may not be sufficient to disqualify the study, they need to be kept in mind, particularly if a second study is identified that does not have these issues.

Is the design of the study internally consistent? Yes. A review of the validation criteria included in the CAT does not reveal any significant problems. As an aside, a single evaluator eliminates any internal validation issues but does present a potential problem for generalization of the findings, particularly if the interpretation of the patella instability test is highly subjective.

What do the results of the study show? Using the method of preponderance of evidence, this study suggests that a negative patellar instability test is highly reliable, assuming that the prevalence of patellar dislocation in the selected population is approximately 50%. Under these conditions, a negative test will miss no more than 3% of patients with 95% certainty and will miss 1% of patients on average. Interestingly enough, the test will miss no more than 5% of patients on average if the prevalence of patellar dislocation was lowered to 18% and no more than 10% of patients would be missed with 95% certainty.

From the other side, patients with anterior knee pain, joint instability, and a positive test have at least an 82% probability of patellar dislocation (with 95% certainty) and an 89% probability on average. Again this assumes a prevalence of approximately 50% in the sample population.

Final conclusion: *In patients with anterior knee pain and knee instability, the patellar instability test is a sensitive and specific test for patellar dislocation.* Since the patient has a positive test, I would tell him that it is very likely that he has a dislocation of his kneecap. Since I am not an orthopedic surgeon, at this point I would explain the need for orthopedic consultation to further discuss treatment options.

Let's see how our students did with a clinical question of prognosis.

CAT 3

Turrentine MA, Ramirez MM. Recurrence of group B streptococci colonization in subsequent pregnancy. *Obstet Gynecol* 2008; 112:259–264.

Patient

A 24-year-old G2P1 at 35 weeks who had group B streptococcus isolated from her vagina (GBS+) during her last pregnancy and received antibiotics intrapartum wants to know the likelihood that she will require treatment again.

Question

What is the likelihood of recurrent colonization with Group B Streptococci (GBS) in women who were GBS+ in their previous pregnancy?

Search Strategies

Search Engine: PubMed
Database: Medline
Key Words: Group B Streptococci, recurrence
Filters: None

Study Summary

Study Type: Case control
Study Population: 102 women who were GBS+ in their index pregnancy and had singleton, uncomplicated second pregnancies.
Intervention: None
Comparison: 102 women who were GBS− in their index pregnancy and had singleton, uncomplicated second pregnancies.
Outcome Measures: Second-pregnancy GBS cultures

Clinical Bottom Lines

1. 54/102 (53%) GBS+ mothers and 15/102 (15%) GBS− mothers were culture positive during the second pregnancy.
2. The rate ratio (GBS+/GBS−) is 3.6 (SD = .34)

Validity Criteria

1. *Was a cohort of patients assembled early in the course of the disease?* This was a case-control study, in which the study populations were selected from all of the women at a single clinic who had two consecutive vaginal deliveries with GBS cultures available.

2. *Do the patients represent population-based samples?* Since this study included all patients at the clinic for which the required data were available and had reasonable inclusion/exclusion criteria, it does represent a population-based sample.

3. *Was the outcome for the study well defined and was follow-up adequate?* The outcome of positive vs. negative cultures was well defined, and follow-up was adequate since the endpoint was culture results of the next pregnancy. The study could have perhaps been improved by following further future pregnancies, but this was not an objective.

4. *Were risk factors shown to be independent?* No, since a multivariate analysis was not performed.

5. *Was the logistic model derived from the risk factor analysis validated in a second cohort of patients?* No. This is a weakness of the current study.

Prepared by Brian Canfield

Do the results of this study apply to the index patient? Assuming that this is a singleton, uncomplicated pregnancy, yes. Mothers who are GBS+ during pregnancy receive antimicrobial therapy during labor and delivery, so this study is particularly relevant to this patient.

Is the design of the study valid for the question raised? Yes, but with qualifications. The best design would have been a prospective, observational study where identification of a variety of potential risk factors would have occurred at the time of enrollment. Economic status, maternal age, parity, and many other factors have been associated with an increased risk of GBS colonization and subsequent neonatal disease. In addition, a prospective cohort study will provide information on the prevalence of subsequent colonization in this patient population, a critical factor in determining the predictive values for prior colonization as well as other risk factors. The outcome data from a case control can be expressed as a likelihood ratio (in fact, that is the only way data from this type of study can be expressed); the design, as noted earlier, is subject to recall and selection bias.

Is the design of the study internally consistent? The conduct of the study is appropriate for a case-control study. Although the study lacks validation, this really looks at a single risk factor, prior colonization, and does not attempt to develop a clinical prediction rule.

What do the results of the study show? By preponderance of evidence, we can say with 95% certainty that a woman who was colonized with GBS during a prior pregnancy is at least 3.04 times as likely to be colonized during a subsequent pregnancy than a women who was not colonized during the index pregnancy. This statement would also form the conclusion for this study. I would explain to the patient that there is large likelihood that she will have to be treated during her next pregnancy.

What about a clinical prediction rule? I gave the following clinical scenario to fourth-year students as part of their advanced experience in medical decision making:

> A 22-year-old, previously healthy college student is brought to the emergency room after sustaining a head injury in a campus touch football game. Witnesses state that he struck his head on the ground and was unconscious for "a few minutes." He has no known allergies and takes no medications. He denies headache, vomiting, or seizure after the injury. At the time he is seen in the emergency room, he is alert and oriented. His Glasgow coma score (GCS) is 15, d he is without focal neurological deficit on physical examination. Should a CAT scan of the head be performed?

CAT 4

Smits M, et al. Predicting intracranial traumatic findings on computed tomography in patients with minor head injury: The CHIP prediction rule. *Ann Intern Med* 2007; 146:397.

Patient

A 22-year-old previously healthy patient who presents following minor head injury and loss of consciousness

Question

In a patient with minor head injury and loss of consciousness who denies headache, vomiting, and seizure and presents with a GCS of 15 and no neurological deficits, should a computed tomography (CT) scan be performed?

Search Strategies

Search Engine: PubMed
Database: Clinical Queries, Clinical Search Strategy: Clinical Prediction Guides
Key Words: CT, head trauma
Filters: English

Study Summary

Study Type: Prospective, observational study
Study Population: 3181 adult patients (greater than or equal to age 16) with minor head injury with a GCS of 13–14 or a GCS of 15 and at least one

risk factor. Patients presented within 24 hours of blunt head injury. Risk factors were history of loss of consciousness, short-term memory deficit, amnesia for the event, seizure, vomiting, severe headache, intoxication with alcohol or drugs, use of anticoagulants or history of coagulopathy, external evidence of injury above clavicles, and neurological deficits

Intervention: CT scan

Comparison: None

Outcome Measures: Any intracranial traumatic CT finding and neurosurgical intervention

Clinical Bottom Lines

1. A CT is indicated if one major criterion is present:
   Pedestrian or cyclist vs. car
   Ejected from vehicle
   Vomiting
   Posttraumatic amnesia ≥4 hours
   Clinical signs of skull fx
   GCS <15
   GCS deterioration ≥2 points (1 hr post presentation)
   Hx of anticoagulant therapy
   Posttraumatic seizure
   Age ≥60 years

   A CT is indicated if two minor criteria are present:
   Fall from any elevation
   Persistent amterograde amnesia (any defect in short-term memory)
   Contusion of skull
   Neurologic deficit
   Loss of consciousness
   GCS deterioration of 1 point (1 hr post presentation)
   Age 40–60 years

2. The CHIP rule has a sensitivity/specificity of 100%/23% for detecting neurosurgical intervention and 96%/25% for detecting intracranial traumatic findings.
   a. With a prevalence of .5% for neurosurgical interventions in 3181 patients the *average* negative predictive value is 100% (LR− = 23 [approx.])
   b. With a prevalence of 7.6% for intracranial trauma in 3181 patients, the *average* negative predictive value is 97.7% (LR− = 6.25)

Validity Criteria

The patient population was well defined. The risk factors that were selected were shown to have a predictive effect in other clinical predictive rules, the New Orleans Criteria (NOC) and the Canadian CT Head Rule (CCHR). All patients were assessed for each risk factor; however, one limitation of this study was that there was a high proportion of patients with at least one unknown variable, mostly because of the difficulty in obtaining a reliable history of loss of consciousness and amnesia.

The data were collected prospectively. The source of the patients was university hospital emergency departments. There is a clearly defined diagnostic outcome of any intracranial traumatic finding (including all neurocranial traumatic findings except for isolated linear skill fractures). Any neurosurgical intervention contingent to the initial CT was a secondary outcome measure. The sample size is large enough to delineate an affected and unaffected group. This study required at least 10 events of intracranial CT findings for each variable. There were 25 variables, so 250 events were required. They needed to include 3125 patients given that the incidence of traumatic findings on CT was 8%–10%. A univariate analysis was performed and the continuous variables of age, amnesia, and GCS showed a linear association with the probability of intracranial traumatic CT findings. A multivariable logistic regression analysis was also performed.

A simple prediction model consisting of 10 major factors and 8 minor factors was developed. Internal validation showed the sensitivity for the neurosurgical intervention was 100% with a specificity of 23% if at least one major or two minor risk factors were present. However, this clinical prediction rule would have missed nine patients with traumatic lesions on CT (sensitivity of 96% and specificity of 25%). It is questionable whether this sensitivity is acceptable for clinical use and whether potentially fatal outcomes could be missed. In this study, the 4% of patients who would have been missed had minor CT findings and did not require any intervention.

This study was not externally validated. An external validation is needed with a different population. Two other clinical prediction rules (NOC and CCHR) have been published and externally validated for CT use in patients with minor head trauma and loss of consciousness. The present study looks at patients with or without loss of consciousness to develop a more widely applicable clinical prediction rule.
Prepared by Kristen Auwarter

Do the results of this study apply to the index patient? He has a history of head trauma, loss of consciousness, and a GCS of 15. These criteria are consistent with those of the patients included in the study.

Is the design of the study valid for the question raised? This is a prospective, cohort study, multicenter in nature. This is the best kind of study for addressing this issue.

Is the design of the study internally consistent? Not completely. Kristen did a great job of identifying most of the problems with this study. A large number of patients were identified and followed through prospectively;

however, the number of patients requiring neurosurgical intervention was still small (17/3181). Both univariate and multivariate analyses were performed. This study derives the clinical prediction rule. Validation is still required. That is a problem. As Kristen notes, two other clinical prediction rules have already been published and validated. As such the use of these other rules should supersede this rule until a validation study is published.

What do the results of the study show? Using the formula from Chapter 6, the standard error surrounding the negative predictive value for neurosurgical intervention is .0018 such that we can say with 95% certainty that the error rate for this model is no more than .3%. This phenomenal negative predictive value is the result of the rarity of neurosurgical interventions, not the strength of the rule. As such, it is essential that this part of the rule be applied only to a population of patients with a comparable a priori risk of injury requiring neurosurgical intervention. Similarly, we can say with 95% certainty that the risk of missing intracranial trauma of any kind is no more than 2.7% when this rule is applied. We can summarize the findings of this study as: *Given the caveat that this clinical rule has not been validated, among head trauma patients the application of this rule to determine whether a CT scan should be performed to identify intracranial head trauma will result in an error rate of no more than 2.7%.* What to do is an interesting decision. Some physicians and patients would be uncomfortable with a maximum error rate of 2.7%, particularly if they believe that there is no significant risk to CT scans. I would tell the patient that in large populations of patients with the same problem, the chances that a CT scan will find something that requires neurosurgery are very small,. One option would be a re-examination in 24–48 hours if the patient did not feel better and to see a physician right away if things became worse. The other option would be to perform the scan and if it's negative, the same follow up rules would apply. My choice would be ＿＿＿＿＿. You can fill in the blank.

One of our students encountered a 17-year-old female with a 2-week history of fever and no predisposing factors or localizing signs.

CAT 5

Vanderschueren S, et al. From prolonged febrile illness to fever of unknown origin. *Arch Intern Med* 2003; 163:1033.

Patient

A 17-year-old female with persistent fever for 2 weeks.

Question

What is the differential diagnosis of a prolonged fever of unknown origin in a 17-year-old female with a fever for over 2 weeks?

Search Strategies

Search Engine: PubMed
Database: Clinical Study Category
Key Words: Fever of unknown origin
Filters: Etiology

Study Summary

Study Type: Prospective cohort
Study Population: 290 immunocompetent patients between 1990 and 1999 with a febrile illness of uncertain cause
Intervention: None
Comparison: Patients were categorized according to the timing of diagnosis—early diagnosis, intermediate diagnosis, late diagnosis, or no diagnosis.
Outcome Measures: The final diagnosis established at discharge or during follow-up

Clinical Bottom Lines

1. The diagnosis was made early (within 3 days) in 23.1%, intermediate (between 4 and 7 days) in 13.1%, and late (after 7 days) in 30.0%. A final diagnosis was absent in 33.8% of patients.
2. Final diagnoses included noninfectious inflammatory diseases (35.4%), infections (29.7%), and neoplasms (15.1%).
3. The most common inflammatory diseases were connective tissue diseases and vasculitis. The most common connective tissue diseases were adult-onset Still's disease and systemic lupus erythematosus. The most common vasculitis syndrome was giant-cell arteritis.
4. The most common infectious causes were endocarditis and cytomegalovirus.
5. The most common neoplasms were hematological, including non-Hodgkin lymphoma and leukemia.
6. Infection was the most common cause of early diagnosis. Neoplasms tended to be diagnosed later as well as noninfectious inflammatory diseases.
7. Biopsy was the most revealing test, especially in the groups with intermediate or late diagnosis.
8. History and evolution was the most common diagnostic method.

Validity Criteria

1. The patient population was not specific to the patient in question. This study included adults ages 33–65, and the patient was a pediatric patient. The symptomology was similar as this study

included patients with elevated temperature greater than 38.3°C for more than 3 weeks.

2. The study included a large study population of 290 patients. The differential diagnosis of fever of unknown origin is extensive, so large study population is needed.

3. The diagnostic evaluation is not completely described. This study does not describe all the specific elements of the medical history, physical findings, and diagnostic evaluation on each patient. What is described are the diagnostic methods that successfully determined the diagnosis, although they do not indicate which test resulted in which diagnosis. The diagnostic methods are instead categorized by the timing of diagnosis (early, intermediate, late). The authors do state that a minimal diagnostic workup was required and that demographic data, details of history, and findings from physical exam and laboratory and technical investigations were registered in a structured data collection form.

4. The constellation of clinical signs is defined for the sample population. To be included in the final database, patients had to have duration of illness of more than 3 weeks before diagnosis and repeated documented body temperatures exceeding 38.3°C.

5. All of the patients are accounted for diagnostically. One hundred ninety two patients were given a diagnosis, and 98 remained without diagnosis. A number of diagnoses were in the "other" category but were labeled in the footnotes of the diagnostic table.

Prepared by Nicole Dominick

Do the results of this study apply to the index patient? That is a difficult question to answer. When I repeated Nicole's search using "all child" and "comparative studies" as limits and the search term ("differential diagnosis" *or* etiology) in addition to "fever of unknown origin," I found no patient series that included children exclusively. There was one series that looked at infants. I happen to know of three old studies that looked exclusively at children, but the patients averaged 4 years of age.

On the other hand, this study only included individuals who were immunocompetent. The literature is replete with studies of febrile neutropenic patients who have a much different differential diagnosis than normal patients. On that point, I think this study is appropriate.

In the final analysis, I believe that Nicole found the most applicable evidence available. We need to keep in mind that the average age of these patients was much more than 17 years.

Is the design of the study valid for the question raised? Yes. A cohort of patients was assembled and studied forward in time. Often studies of this nature are retrospective and represent a group of patients identified from a database. From a design point of view, this study is of high quality.

Is the design of the study internally consistent? Nicole has done a great job validating this study. She points out that it is not clear that each patient underwent the same clinical evaluation or that a diagnostic protocol was followed. One result of this design flaw is the large percentage of undiagnosed patients. On the other hand, the patients were well described.

What do the results of the study show? As stated in the Clinical Bottom Lines, of those patients with a diagnosis, 35% of patients had an inflammatory disease, 30% had an infection, and 15% had a neoplasm. Approximately one-third of patients did not receive a diagnosis. The most common inflammatory diseases were adult-onset Still disease, lupus erythematosus, and giant-cell arteritis. Infective endocarditis and cytomegalovirus infection were the most common infections, while leukemia and lymphoma were the predominant neoplasms. The data from this study are sufficiently specific that a clinician can easily develop a diagnostic plan for a 17-year-old patient with 3 weeks of fever and a negative workup for common etiologies such as urinary tract infections, sexually transmitted diseases, and sinusitis. Nicole's conclusion for this study: *"The most common causes of fever of unknown origin are connective tissue diseases, vasculitis syndromes, and infections."* Nicole should evaluate the patient for the most common entities on her list. What should she say to her patient? Talking to patients about differential diagnoses is difficult. If you give too much information, the patient may become confused or worried about serious entities with low probabilities. If you give too little information, the patient may feel you are hiding something or that you are unsure. One approach is to delineate the large categories (e.g., infection and immune mediated) and discuss, in general, what types of tests you plan to do (blood tests, imaging tests, etc.). Experts are divided on how to handle things if neoplasia is in the differential diagnosis. I believe you must mention it if you plan on a biopsy or other invasive procedure to rule it out or if you think it is a real possibility.

The first type of study to look to for answers to your therapeutic and diagnostic questions is a meta-analysis. These types of studies have the most power, demonstrate consistency in results across multiple studies, and are viewed by many as the highest quality of evidence for answering clinical questions. In Chapter 11, I presented a meta-analysis that addressed a question of therapeutics. In this chapter I would like to present one that addresses the issue of diagnosis. Consider the following case:

> A 15-year-old girl with a past medical history of an eating disorder is admitted with anemia. She was well and in a residential facility until 2 months prior to admission when she developed sharp, mid-epigastric pain that was relieved with eating. The pain was intermittent. Approximately 2 weeks prior to admission she noted that her stools had become tarry in appearance and sticky. She did not mention this to any of the providers at the facility. Five days prior to admission the abdominal pain worsened and on the day of

admission she complained of dizziness. In the emergency department, she was tachycardic and demonstrated orthostatic changes in
blood pressure. She had mid-epigastric pain to deep palpation and
her stool tested positive for blood. Her hemoglobin was 6 g/L. A
clinical diagnosis of peptic ulcer disease was made. She was trans-
fused and begun on a proton pump inhibitor.

Since most cases of peptic ulcer disease in childhood and adolescence are
associated with *H. pylori* infection, the issue of diagnosis was raised. Since
the gastroenterologists did not think endoscopy was warranted given her
clinical response to transfusion and the absence of blood in her stools
over time, the house staff wondered whether there was another way to
make the diagnosis of *H. pylori* infection. I provided them with the CAT
below.

CAT 6

Gisbert JP, de la Morena F, Abraira V. Accuracy of monoclonal stool antigen test for the diagnosis of *H. pylori* infection: a systematic review and
meta-analysis. *Am J Gastro* 2006; 101:1921–1930.

Patient

A 15-year-old female with acute history of mid-epigastric pain responsive
to proton pump inhibitors and upper gastrointestinal bleeding.

Question

What is the best way to diagnose *H. pylori* infection noninvasively and
without using the urea breath test?

Search Strategies

Search Engine: PubMed systematic review query
Database: Medline
Key Words: *H. pylori*, diagnosis
Filters: English, all child

Study Summary

Study Type: Meta-analysis
Study Population: Studies of stool antigen testing for *H. pylori* in populations of children or adults with suspected peptic ulcer disease
Intervention: Stool assay for *H. pylori* using a monoclonal antibody detection system
Comparison: Gold standard defined by rapid urease test of biopsied material, tissue histology, tissue culture, urea breath test, and/or serology
Outcome Measures: Sensitivity and specificity of stool antigen test with
   gold standard

Clinical Bottom Lines

1. Before treatment studies
   a. The database consisted of 22 studies (2499 patients; mixed adults and children).
   b. The average prevalence rate of infection was .62 (range .28–1.0).
   c. The overall sensitivity was .94 (95% CI: .93–.95). Significant heterogeneity was found and was due to a single outlier.
   d. The overall specificity was .97 (95% CI: .96–.98) Significant heterogeneity was found and was due to a single outlier.
   e. The overall LR+ was 24 (95% CI: 15–41).
   f. The overall LR– was .07 (95% CI: .04–.12).

2. Eradiation studies
   a. The database consisted of 12 studies (957 patients; 94 children).
   b. The average treatment failure rate was .2 (range: 0–.32).
   c. The overall sensitivity was .93 (95% CI: .89–.96) Significant heterogeneity was found and was due to a single outlier.
   d. The overall specificity was .96 (95% CI: .94–.97) Significant heterogeneity was found and was due to a single outlier.
   e. The overall LR+ was 17 (95% CI: 12–23).
   f. The overall LR– was .1 (95% CI: .07–.15).

Validity Criteria

1. *Does the study address a well-defined clinical question?* Yes.
2. *Was a research protocol defined prior to the initiation of the study?* Yes. Also all subset analyses were defined a priori.
3. *Was an exhaustive search made to discover all relevant articles?* Yes. The authors searched the MEDLINE, EMBASE, and Cochrane databases as well as abstracts from the International Workshop of Gastroduodenal Pathology and *H. pylori* up to the year 2005 and the American Digestive Disease Week. Articles in Japanese were excluded.
4. *Was there an accounting of all of the articles?* Yes.
5. *Was a summary table included in the meta-analysis?* Yes.
6. *Was a statistical method used to consolidate the data from all of the studies?* The random effects method was used.
7. *Was a sensitivity analysis performed?* Yes, based on gold standard, adults versus children, and metaregression versus quality scores.
8. *Was publication bias addressed?* No.
9. *Was heterogeneity addressed?* Yes.

Prepared by Stephen Aronoff

Is the design of the study valid for the question raised? The design is a meta-analysis, which is the best form of evidence for a question of diagnosis or treatment. A close review of this article shows that the number of patients included in individual studies ranges from 53 to 378 in the diagnostic studies and 32 to 325 in the eradication studies; the meta-analyses included 2499 patients in the diagnostic analysis and 987 patients in the eradication analysis. The vast increase in sample population results in the narrow confidence intervals of the overall outcomes. This is the major advantage of meta-analysis.

Is the design of the study internally consistent? This study met most of the validation criteria. Inclusion criteria and subset analyses were determined a priori, the authors provided a detailed map of both the search and the fate of the articles found, an appropriate statistical method was used to combine the studies, heterogeneity was addressed, and a sensitivity analysis was performed. The only internal flaw was the failure of the authors to address publication bias.

What do the results of the study show? Let's look at the question of diagnosis first since that is germane to our clinical question. We can use the sensitivity and specificity data to calculate the positive and negative likelihood ratios, but the authors have kindly provided us with that information as well as the prevalence range for the study. The LR+ is 24 with a 95% confidence interval of 15 to 41. From this, we can estimate that the standard deviation is $(24 - 15)/2 = 4.5$. We can calculate that the 90% lower confidence interval is 16.6; $[24 - (1.65 \times 4.5)]$. We *can* say with 95% certainty that patients with a positive stool antigen test have at least 16.6 times greater chance of *H. pylori* infection than those with a negative test because the positive LR addresses the ratio of true positives to false positives; it says nothing about patients with negative tests. We *do* know that .28 (a priori odds = $.28/.72 = .39$) was the *lowest* prevalence rate of *H. pylori* infection in the study. Using the odds expression, we can say with 95% that the posterior odds of being infected with *H. pylori* if the stool antigen test is positive are at least $.39 \times 16.6 = 6.5$. Converting this to a probability, we can finally conclude with 95% certainty that the positive predictive value of the stool antigen test is at least 87% *or* that the error rate of the stool antigen is no more than 13%. This is the worse-case scenario using the lowest prevalence rate of the disease. Using the average prevalence rate of the disease (.62), a similar calculation allows us to say with 95% certainty that the positive predictive value of the stool antigen test is at least 97% *or* that the error rate is no more than 3%. Convince yourself that this last calculation is correct.

From the meta-analysis, the authors note that the overall negative likelihood ratio was .07 with a 95% confidence interval of .04 to .12. These numbers seem wrong compared to the numbers we calculated before. Remember that in Chapter 6, we defined the rate of absence of disease as 1 – prevalence rate. The negative likelihood ratio was defined as specificity/(1 – sensitivity). These authors have chosen to define the negative likelihood ratio as the inverse, (1 – sensitivity/specificity). The product of this value and the actual prevalence rate expressed as odds yields a new, smaller prevalence rate, expressed as odds. Converting this to a probability and subtracting it from 1 gives us the negative predictive value. So here goes:

1. Calculating the 90% *upper* confidence interval as before, we get .12 – .025 = .095.
2. The *highest* prevalence rate among the studies included in the meta-analysis was 1. We obviously can't use that, so let's use the average prevalence rate of .62 and its a priori odds of 1.63.
3. .095 × 1.63 = .15
4. Converting to a probability, .15/(1 + 1.15) = .13

In this case, we can say that the *error* rate in the negative predictive value is no more than 13% and that the negative predictive value is at least 87%. It is coincidental that these values match the error rate and positive predictive value when .28 was used as the prevalence rate. From all of this we can conclude the following: *The stool antigen test for H. pylori is an excellent diagnostic test with an average positive error rate of less than 3% and an average negative error rate of 13%.*

Given this conclusion, I chose to perform the test. What did I tell the patient and her mother? I began by explaining that we needed to rule in or rule out this diagnosis since it would have an impact on therapy (combination anti-infective therapy plus a proton pump inhibitor is currently recommended for *H. pylori* infections). I further explained that a stool test involved less risk and discomfort than endoscopy and that endoscopy was not indicated at this time, since her symptoms had improved. Finally, I explained that while the stool test was not perfect (i.e., a gold standard), it provided enough certainty that we could base both therapeutic and outcome decisions on the test results. I went on to say that if her symptoms recurred or were not eliminated by the therapy we chose based on the stool antigen results, we would want to revisit the issue of endoscopy.

The last CAT I want to address is one of causality. As we discussed in the previous chapter, there are a host of criteria that must be met in order to make a reasonable case for causation. Only rarely will a single article meet all of these criteria. As part of the "Medical Decision Making" course at Temple, I have used the following practica to see whether students have mastered the material relating to causation:

In 2003, an outbreak of a severe respiratory illness occurred in China, other parts of the Far East, and in Canada. Severe acute respiratory syndrome (SARS) was rapidly investigated by the world health community. Identify a single article that contributes to our understanding of the etiology of this disorder and analyze its validity in CAT format.

CAT 7

Drosten C, et al. Identification of a novel coronavirus in patients with severe acute respiratory syndrome. *N Engl J Med* 2003 May 15; 348(20):1967-1976.

Patient

Looking at those patients afflicted with severe acute respiratory syndrome during the outbreak in Vietnam in 2002.

Question

What is the etiologic agent causing SARS?

Search Strategies

Search Engine: PubMed
Database: PubMed
Key Words: Etiology of severe acute respiratory syndrome
Filters: Publication date from 2002 to 2008, Humans, English, Core clinical journals, All Adults: 19+ years

Study Summary

Study Type: Research study where clinical specimens from patients with SARS were searched for unknown viruses with the use of cell cultures and molecular techniques.

Study Population: Index patient plus two contacts. A total of 49 specimens from 18 patients with suspected or probable SARS, according to the WHO case definition, and from 21 healthy contact persons were sampled between March 5 and March 27, 2003, during the SARS epidemic in Hanoi, Vietnam.

Intervention: None

Comparison: A total of 54 stool samples from patients in Germany were available as controls.

Outcome Measures: (1) Polymerase chain reaction (PCR) to test for *Mycoplasma pneumoniae, Chlamydia pneumoniae,* human cytomegalovirus, adenoviruses, respiratory syncytial virus, parainfluenzavirus types 1, 2, 3, and 4, Hendra virus, Nipah virus, human metapneumovirus, influenzaviruses A and B, rhinovirus, and human coronavirus strains OC43 and 229E, herpesviruses, arenaviruses, bunyaviruses, enteroviruses, alphaviruses, flaviviruses, filoviruses, and paramyxoviruses; (2) Searched for homologies to known sequences using the nucleotide or translated database of the Basic Local Alignment Search Tool (BLAST) at http://www.ncbi.nlm.nih.gov:80/BLAST/.

Clinical Bottom Lines

1. Paramyxovirus-like particles were seen in throat swabs and sputum samples from the index patient by electron microscopy, but the particles were scarce and PCR was negative.
2. *C. pneumonia* was not detected by PCR or antigen ELISA in sputum of the index patient on day 9, but day 11 electron microscopy of bronchoalveolar lavage cells showed intracellular bacterial infection.
3. After 6 days of incubation, a cytopathic effect was seen on Vero-cell cultures inoculated with sputum obtained from the index patient from which 20 distinct DNA fragments were obtained and sequenced. A translated BLAST search showed homology to coronavirus amino acid sequence, indicating that a coronavirus had been isolated.
4. The isolate was compared with one obtained by the Centers for Disease Control and Prevention (CDC), and both sequences were 100% identical.
5. Diagnostic PCR assays were established by designing a nested set of primers within the BNI-1 fragment. The outer set of primers detected the virus in clinical specimens from the index patients and Contact 1, who also had clinical signs of SARS.
6. Further specimens from patients with probable and suspected SARS and well as healthy contacts of patients affected by the SARS epidemic in Hanoi, Vietnam were tested by nested PCR assays targeting the CDC and BNI-1 fragments. The prevalence of the virus was 100% among patients with probable cases of SARS and 23% among suspected cases, and the virus was not detected at all in healthy contacts.

Validity Criteria

1. There is a strong exposure–outcome relationship. In this study, the subjects were identified by the signs and symptoms of SARS (fever, dry cough, dyspnea, headache, and hypoxemia, lymphopenia and mildly elevated aminotransferase levels, death from progressive respiratory failure due to alveolar damage) and were compared to healthy controls that did not show signs or symptoms of SARS. The probable cases of SARS showed evidence of a coronavirus infection, while healthy controls did not.
2. The association was consistent in the study. The virus was identified in the index patient by one obtained separately from the CDC and in further studies of suspected cases of SARS. However, this study does not include any other patients besides the ones afflicted in the Vietnam epidemic.
3. The exposure cannot be temporally related to the outcome, because the virus was identified after the symptoms developed.

4. The agent was identified in patients with the disease via PCR and serologic evidence was found in a number of other individuals with the disease. However, it was not proven in this study that the coronavirus is necessary for SARS, but it is sufficient to cause SARS.
5. The association between a coronavirus and SARS is biologically plausible since other coronaviruses have been known to cause minor respiratory illnesses.

Conclusion: *A novel coronavirus may be the etiologic agent of severe acute respiratory syndrome (SARS)*
Prepared by Nicole Dominick

Nicole has done a terrific job of finding appropriate evidence and validating it. Since the types of studies that address causality are myriad, determining whether the study contributes to our understanding of causality of a disease entity should use the criteria detailed in the previous chapter as a road map for validation.

The exposure–outcome relationship hinges on the fact that a coronavirus was isolated from patients with clinically defined SARS but not from those without clinical disease. Does this scenario sound like the findings between Cat scratch disease and *Afipia felis?* The finding that infected patients had demonstrable antibody to the virus supports this point. A coronavirus as the cause of SARS is also biologically plausible. These are the main findings of the paper. Nicole correctly points out the other weaknesses of the paper.

I realize this last chapter may have been tedious. My goals were to demonstrate how the CAT format can be used to summarize clinical evidence and how facile third-year medical students can be in finding and validating evidence. The CAT is a wonderful tool for education at all levels of training. As you can see, I have used it extensively in the online course taught at Temple to assess student mastery of the skills of medical decision making.

15

DEVELOPING A
PLAN FOR LIFELONG
EDUCATION

Congratulations. If you have stuck it out this far, you now have the skills to find, validate, critically analyze, and apply the clinical literature to the care of your patients. After all of this work, it would be a shame not to use and develop these skills on a daily basis.

As health care providers, we are ethically (and legally) bound to provide the best care to our patients at all times. Since the database of clinical studies is constantly expanding with thousands of new studies added on a regular basis, given these expectations (not to mention the licensure laws in most states), health care professionals have both statutory and personal requirements for ongoing education. How to enhance clinical knowledge given the ever-increasing demands on providers' and trainees' time is a huge problem. A combination of attending continuing medical education (CME) lectures or courses and reading the latest journals in free time (usually between 2 and 4 a.m.!) is the method selected by most. Since you have just about completed this book, a third option for self-education should be apparent: identifying and validating the evidence for clinical issues that occur in your daily practice. Let's examine these three avenues for self-education and see how they can fit together.

WHAT CONFERENCES AND CONTINUING MEDICAL EDUCATION ACTIVITIES DO I NEED AND WHY?

Most states have a minimum number of instructional hours required for re-licensure as a physician or professional health care provider. For physicians, a fixed number of these hours must be in American Medical Association Category 1, defined as approved programs meeting a fixed number of requirements and sponsored by a hospital, medical school, or other organizational body. Some articles in journals also provide category 1 CME activity. Attending CME lectures and classes are the most common methods of self-learning, since these types of activities are usually tied to category 1 hours. Many community hospitals offer 1 or 2 hours per week of approved CME activities. Sponsored lectures by outside speakers or lectures presented by medical staff are often presented in a grand rounds format. The topics vary and may cover issues germane to internal medicine, surgery, pediatrics, OB/GYN, and other specialties represented at the hospital. A major drawback to these types of rounds is applicability. For example, a pediatrician listening to an update talk on the management of acute myocardial infarction will receive credit for attendance but is unlikely to gain any information useful to her practice. Academic medical centers present hundreds of hours of CME activities each week. Grand rounds are offered weekly in each major specialty and subspecialty; case conferences, journal clubs, and other CME activities are also provided. Unfortunately, not everyone has ready access or has the time to spend going to an academic medical center several times a week for CME activities.

Many professional organizations, hospitals, and universities offer 1–5-day-long CME programs. These programs may be topic driven (e.g., care of the elderly patient or care of the patient with asthma), updates, or review courses for board examination. Programs associated with annual meetings of specialty organizations have robust agendas with new research presentations, topical discussions, "meet the professor" sessions, as well as panel discussions of "hot topics."

Given all of these choices and the limitations of time and money, what objectives should drive a health care provider's decisions? One criterion is how directly does the material in the CME activity address issues that are confronted in the practitioner's daily dealings with patients. In the Preface, I stated that my practice is limited to children with infectious diseases. Naturally, the vast majority of the activities I choose address pediatric infectious disease topics or topics in general pediatrics. I was asked to serve as team physician to my son's Pop Warner football team recently, so I chose to spend some of my CME time at activities focused on the pediatric athlete. Many physicians I know who have relatives with a medical problem outside of their fields may chose to learn more about that disease. In general, the topic should be of interest to you so it serves some purpose other than meeting a statutory obligation for CME hours. I attend at least one CME activity each week offered at the hospital. I also like to attend at least one "away" CME activity each year. I usually choose a national meeting for one of my professional organizations. Many people I know in private practice will attend their annual academy meetings. Not only do these meetings provide CME hours, but they are a good way to catch up on issues facing practitioners in the field and to catch up with old friends.

Attending lectures or classes are not the only Category 1 CME activities. With the development of the Internet and secure online interactions, most of the subspecialty boards offer online CME activities. For example, the American Board of Pediatrics offers a decision skills self-assessment examination on their website. Successful completion of this exam is worth 15 category 1 CME hours. Other self-assessment examinations are available annually in all of the pediatric subspecialty areas. Many journals also offer a category 1 hour for reading an article and submitting the answers to a short quiz.

Keep in mind that these types of CME activities, while informative, are designed to meet a statutory obligation for licensure. The applicability of these activities to patient care is variable, the timing of these activities to issues that arise clinically is random, and the validity of the information presented at many of these activities is not controllable since most presentations represent conclusions drawn by a third party, the speaker. Overall, CME activities should comprise only a small percentage of a practitioner's annual educational time.

SHOULD I SUBSCRIBE TO JOURNALS AND WHICH ONES SHOULD I GET?

The preeminent role "keeping up with the journals" plays in the lifelong educational plan for most health care providers is overrated. Subscribing to three or four journals and reading them cover to cover (or reading the abstracts cover to cover) is a complete waste of time. The successful lifelong student is selective both in the journals read and the articles within those journals that are read.

Let's start with the journals. As was the case with the discussion on CME activities, the most important criterion that should be applied to journal selection is impact on practice. You should pick journals and journal articles that are going to change the way you practice medicine. Unless you have a specific interest in basic science research, the journals you choose should focus on translational research. All of the journals should be peer reviewed, that is, all articles printed in these (and for that matter all of the journals we will be discussing) are reviewed by a panel of experts before the decision to print or reject an article is made. While the basis for these decisions may vary from journal to journal, appropriateness of the study for inclusion in the particular journal, study design, and attention to subject rights are some of the criteria used by most publications. You need to select journals from each of two groups.

General medical journals print articles addressing all specialties of medicine. Examples of some of these journals are *Journal of the American Medical Association (JAMA)*, *British Medical Journal*, *Canadian Medical Association Journal*, *The Lancet*, and *The New England Journal of*

Medicine. Each of these journals has a long history of publication and is well regarded by physicians and researchers alike. Because of the high standards for publication and the broad readership of these journals, authors of clinical studies prefer to publish their highest quality work here. I have subscribed to *The New England Journal of Medicine* since I was a medical student. Although my field of interest is pediatrics and pediatric infectious diseases, I often finding something of clinical use in this journal. I am sure the same can be said for the other journals. I suggest you subscribe to one.

Specialty and subspecialty journals print articles of interest to a narrower, more focused audience. Each medical or surgical specialty organization and many subspecialty organizations sponsor a peer-reviewed publication. In my world the journal *Pediatrics* is the principal journal sponsored by the American Academy of Pediatrics. The journal contains articles of interest to general and subspecialty pediatricians alike. The journal also is the primary source for policy statements and guidelines endorsed by the Academy. Every American pediatrician should subscribe to this journal. Other examples include *Annals of Internal Medicine* (The American College of Physicians) and *Journal of the American College of Surgeons* (The American College of Surgeons).

Subspecialists should subscribe to the appropriate subspecialty journals as well. Since I am a pediatric infectious disease physician, I also subscribe to *The Pediatric Infectious Disease Journal* (Pediatric Infectious Disease Society) and *Clinical Infectious Diseases* (Infectious Disease Society of America). Other subspecialists or those with subspecialty interests should identify those journals associated with their particular subspecialty organizations.

Is a subscription really necessary? Subscriptions to many of these journals are a perquisite of society membership. Except for *The New England Journal of Medicine*, all of my other journal subscriptions were included in the dues for the different societies that I have joined. If you have online access to the journals you want to review regularly, then a subscription may not be necessary. In any case, online access to the most recent issues as well as archived issues is desirable.

When I receive a new issue of any journal, I review the table of contents. When I find an article of interest, I approach it as outlined in Chapter 2. I look first for the hypothesis tested and decide whether I believe it addresses a clinically relevant problem. I move on to the Methods section, paying close attention to the patient population, primary outcome, and study design. Finally, I look at the Results section to decide whether they are clinically significant. I will check my impression of the clinical bottom line of the paper with the abstract to see if they coincide. If not, I may go back to read sections of the paper in detail. I rarely read an entire paper (I usually skip the Discussion). This, of course, is up to you, but it should take no longer than 5 minutes to review a new journal article. I also like to scan the editorials and commentaries for interesting points of view or comments on current medical events. In general, I spend no more than 15% of the time I allocate to self-education with current literature.

WHAT IS THE ROLE OF "PATIENT-DIRECTED" READING IN SELF-EDUCATION?

By now it should be obvious to you that I believe that the vast majority of the time spent in self-education should be spent on patient-directed reading. Identifying the issue that brings a patient to your attention and identifying, validating, and applying the evidence that you find are the best bargains yet in medical education. Not only does it allow you to identify "best practices" for your patients, but you learn something new and you get to apply your new knowledge immediately. As you use these skills more and more, the time needed to find and validate evidence becomes vanishingly small. Finally, understanding the evidence that supports a particular approach or therapy in patient care allows you to identify weaknesses of current approaches and areas to look for in future research. A great example of this happened while I was writing this book. As you remember from the chapter on guidelines, the entire question of imaging children with first urinary tract infections was called into question based on the low yield of tests and the questionable value of prophylactic antibiotics in this patient population. As I was scanning the table of contents of *The New England Journal of Medicine*, I came across the following article: Antibiotic prophylaxis and recurrent urinary tract infection in children (*NEJM* 2009; 361:1748). As you can imagine, I read the article and came across information that may change the way I manage patients. What did I find? Read it and decide for yourself!

HOW DO I GET ACCESS TO JOURNALS BEYOND THE ONES I SUBSCRIBE TO?

Free and open access to the text of journal articles is becoming more prevalent. Any article funded by the National Institutes of Health must be freely available. Links to these articles accompany the abstracts that are published on PubMed. PubMed Central is a huge repository of articles that can be accessed free. BioMed Central is another leading provider of free content. Clicking on these links from PubMed will give you the complete text from any of 250 journals published under their auspices. HighWire press is another free source for journal articles.

A large number of articles are available through the 725 journals listed with Wolters Kluwer/Ovid. This is a pay-for-view service where you can make arrangements to pay for an individual article or subscribe to the service.

The easiest way to access full-text articles online is through an affiliation with a large medical library. Most teaching hospitals with residency programs and all medical schools have extensive libraries. Along with the online access to the subscribed journals, these institutions also participate in other online services, such as Ovid. These services, along with the hardcopy stacks housed in the brick-and-mortar facilities, give you access to almost every reference you will ever need. For those journals that are unavailable, interlibrary loan services can usually provide copies.

Whatever combination of activities you chose, remember the goal of self-education: to provide the highest quality of care to your patients based on the best evidence available. If you incorporate your new skills into your day-to-day patient care activities, I'm sure you will see that finding and using the evidence will become second nature and your patients will appreciate the confidence and candor in their interactions with you.

A FINAL THOUGHT

Over the course of a typical academic year, I will review several hundred independent CATs submitted by third- and fourth-year medical students. On occasion, a student will submit a particularly interesting one. In these cases I like to ask the student some details about the patient or how the evidence was provided to the team. One episode illustrates, at least for me, the real value of asking questions and searching the literature for evidence. The article submitted by the student was a meta-analysis of octreotide therapy in patients undergoing subtotal pancreatectomy. The interesting point about this case was the finding in the meta-analysis that the mortality among octreotide recipients was significantly higher than among those in the placebo group, suggesting that this agent was relatively contraindicated in this clinical setting. When I asked the student about how he came to ask this question, his e-mail response was electric! The senior members of the team caring for the patient believed that octreotide was fully indicated in this population. I don't know the providers' response when the student presented this information, but I will always remember the student's response to my query: "I never thought that 20 minutes in the library with a computer, printer, and copying machine could have such a dramatic impact on patient care." In the end, however you choose to use your newly found skills, always remember the first rule of clinical practice: *primum non nocere!*

16

TEACHING MEDICAL DECISION MAKING

This book has its roots in the "Evidence-Based Medicine" course that I have taught to third-year medical students at Temple University over the past 6 years. When I first came to Temple, I used my position as Chairman of the Department of Pediatrics to incorporate the elements of evidence-based medicine into the 6-week pediatric core clerkship. I was quickly informed by the clerkship director that teaching the elements of evidence-based medicine in the clerkship severely limited lecture time needed to cover the core curriculum in pediatrics. The next evolution spread the elements of evidence-based medicine over the pediatric and family medicine core clerkships. This approach was severely limited by scheduling issues, since the two clerkships could not be consistently conjoined in time.

At this point, I approached the Associate Dean for Medical Education who agreed to give evidence-based medicine course status. Since I wanted students to be able to directly apply medical decision-making skills to patient care, I believed the introduction of this material was most appropriate during the third year of our medical school curriculum when students began clinical rotations. This approach presented two problems. First, the Liaison Committee for Medical Education (LCME) standards dictate that each student must have a comparable experience across regional campus sites. Since Temple had multiple sites where students rotated, a method of course delivery was needed to meet this requirement. Second, since lecture time within each clinical clerkship was at a premium and was slotted differently by each specialty, didactic lectures would have to be given at multiple times across rotations, if they could be arranged at all.

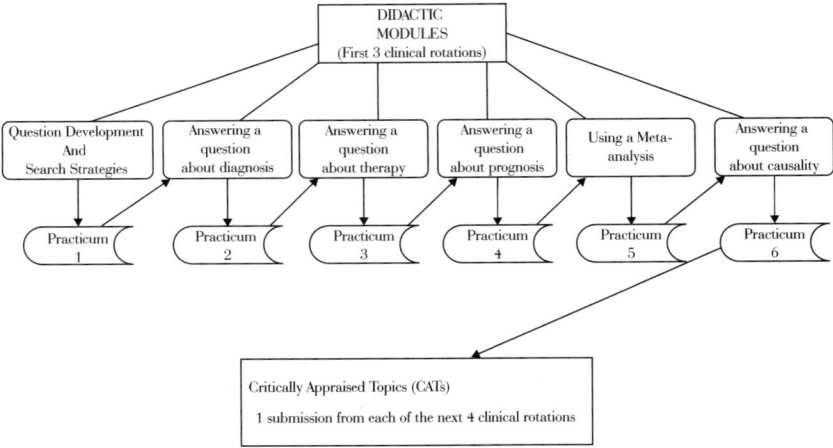

Figure 16-1. Schematic of online course run concurrent with core clerkships. (Reprinted with permission from Aronoff SC, et. al. *Teaching and learning in medicine*, in publication.)

Finally, to provide uniform instruction across all of the specialties and sites would require a huge project in faculty education. All of these problems were addressed by delivering the curriculum online.

As shown in Figure 16-1, the curriculum was divided into six modules, each with an online didactic section. Each student submitted a practicum at the completion of each module to one of five faculty members, who were familiar with the curriculum and trained in evidence-based medicine. Each practicum consisted of a clinical scenario with a directed question. For the second practicum, students were provided with the citation and all evaluated the same evidence. Subsequent exercises required the students to find their own evidence. Following completion of the six modules, each student was required to submit an independent critically appraised topic (CAT) based on a clinical question that was raised during the rotation (Chapter 14).

In 2009, the course was expanded into the last year of medical school. Three modules (advanced clinical trials, clinical prediction rules, and differential diagnosis) were added along with appropriate practica and use of the online faculty mentors. Three independent CATs were also required. Examples of student CATS are included in Chapter 14.

DEVELOPING STUDENT PRACTICA

Developing exercises for each module of the course is central to the learning process. Not only does this provide an opportunity for the student to apply newly gained knowledge in a controlled, favorable situation, it provides feedback to the instructor regarding the student's mastery of the material. In the Temple online course, all practica are clinically based. To develop new practica, I usually start with the evidence. Since it is critical that beginners use studies of the highest quality, I try to pick a high-quality, recently published article that addresses a common issue in medical practice. I usually stumble across these articles in my daily use of the literature to solve my own clinical problems or through scanning of the table of contents of new journals that cross my desk. However you find them, articles should *(1)* address a simple but important clinical question, *(2)* come to a clinically significant conclusion, *(3)* meet most if not all of the validation criteria for the given topic, *(4)* be easy to find in a search using PubMed; and *(5)* be available to the student online.

For example, let's assume the target article is the following: Monto AS, et al. Comparative efficacy of inactivated and live attenuated influenza vaccine. *N Engl J Med* 2009; 361:1260–1267. In this study, the authors compared patients (aged 18 to 49) who received live attenuated or inactivated vaccine during the 2007–2008 influenza season; both preparations contained the same virus strains. The primary outcome was the incidence of flu-like illness confirmed by culture or polymerase chain reaction (PCR) for three groups: placebo recipients; inactivated virus recipients; and live, attenuated virus recipients. The study shows significant differences in protection between the two vaccine preparations.

1. *What clinical question does the article address?* This study addresses a question of therapy (in its broadest sense): "In a group of healthy adults aged 18 to 49, is the live, attenuated influenza vaccine (LAV) as effective as the inactivated vaccine (IV) in preventing symptomatic, culture or PCR proven episodes of influenza?"

2. *Does this article come to a clinically significant conclusion?* The infection rate among LAV recipients was 6.9% and among IV recipients was 3.4%. The rate ratio was 2.2; 95% of the data supported an infection rate among LAV recipients that was at least 83% higher than that of IV recipients. On average, 24 subjects would have to receive IV in order to prevent one infection that would have occurred with LAV.

3. *Does the article meet most of the validation criteria required for a study of this kind?* Yes (see Chapter 5).

4. *Is the study easy to find by searching MEDLINE via PubMed?* Using the PubMed search engine, the search string "influenza immunization" AND live AND attenuated along with the filters "Humans," "clinical trial," and "all adult" yields 24 references. When placed in order of publication, the target article is first. There were at least three other articles of similar design and of equal quality. I have found it useful to review these articles as well, since these studies are valid evidence for the question at hand and may be submitted by students.

5. *Is the article available online? The New England Journal of Medicine* is available to our students online.

Developing a clinical scenario is the next step. Each scenario needs to be realistic. Provide enough information so that the student can not only identify the category of question raised by the scenario (therapy, diagnosis, etc.) but also can generate a question with sufficient detail so the search will return a manageable number of citations as well as the target citation. The scenario also needs to be appropriate for the level of the learner. What should the scenario look like for third-year medical students beginning clinical rotations? Consider the following:

A 36-year-old previously healthy man comes to the family practice clinic for an annual physical examination. As part of your health maintenance guidance, you ask him if he has received flu shots in the past. He states that he has but some of his friends avoided the shot last year by getting a nasal spray. He asks whether the shot (inactivated vaccine) is as good as the nasal spray (live, attenuated vaccine).

Students at this level may not know that two different types of vaccine exist. This fact needs to be incorporated into the scenario.

STUDENT'S RESPONSE TO THE PRACTICA

At the end of this course, I expect each third-year student to be able to generate an independent question from cases seen during clerkships and to generate a CAT that addresses that question. I try to structure the practica in such a way that the student's responses increase in complexity. For the first practicum, I limit the student's response to the generation of a searchable question, elaboration of a search strategy, and the listing of one citation that answers the question. For the next practicum, I supply the student with the article and ask specific questions that walk the student through the components of a CAT. By the third practicum, I expect the students to find the evidence on their own and to report it in CAT format. Throughout the didactic portion of the course, the clinical questions are designed so that each student has an opportunity to find, assess, and validate at least one study addressing each of the topics presented in the course.

FACULTY–STUDENT FEEDBACK AND COURSE COMPLETION

The didactic material with the associated practica is structured to complete five of the topics in the third year and the remaining topics in the fourth year of medical school. The third year of medical school at Temple consists of eight 6-week blocks of time. Students are given three blocks to complete the didactic material and are expected to turn in four independent CATS by the end of the year. Each practicum and CAT is submitted to a faculty member by e-mail. Errors that are identified in each submission are brought to the student's attention. Students are expected to correct the errors and resubmit the material. The fourth-year consists of twelve 4-week blocks. The first three blocks of the fourth year are dedicated to the completion of the didactic material; four independent CATs are required to complete the course. Successful completion of all practica and CATS is required for course completion. At Temple, both the third- and fourth-year courses are pass/fail.

SAMPLE CLINICAL SCENARIOS

Here are some clinical scenarios that I have used over the years. The questions are straightforward and the answers are not hard to find. I am not giving the answers! Try this yourself and see if you can answer them.

1. A 2-month-old infant with a history of prematurity (26 weeks estimated gestational age), respiratory distress syndrome, and bronchopulmonary dysplasia requiring ongoing oxygen therapy presents to the clinic in November. Because of the risk of respiratory syncytial virus infection (bronchiolitis), you wonder if passively immunizing him with antibody against the virus will prevent or reduce the risk of infection and its complications.

2. A 2-year-old African American child is brought to the emergency room with the acute onset of pain and swelling in the hands and feet. His past medical history is remarkable for five prior episodes of similar nature. The child's mother relates that a hemoglobin screen performed at birth was positive for hemoglobin S disease. Aside from tachycardia, pallor, and swelling of the hands and feet, the physical examination is normal. Initial laboratory values reveal a hemoglobin of 5.5 g/dL and a WBC of 25,000 cells/mm^3. The child is admitted and hydrated. During the hospitalization, the mother expresses deep concern regarding strokes and death from sickle cell disease.

3. In 2003, an outbreak of a severe respiratory illness occurred in China, other parts of the Far East, and in Canada. Severe acute respiratory syndrome (SARS) was rapidly investigated by the world health community. Identify a single article that contributes to our understanding of the etiology of this disorder and analyze its validity in CAT format (see Chapter 14 for the associated student CAT).

4. A 10-year-old child comes to your office with a 1-week history of diarrhea. She recently returned from a 2-week trip to India. The diarrhea began while she was in India. No other family members are sick. Two days ago, she was seen in a local emergency room for evaluation of diarrhea. A stool culture was performed and yielded *Shigella dysenteriae* type I. The organism

was sensitive to ciprofloxacin. You want to treat for 5 days, but the family has no insurance and has to pay for the medication themselves. Are 3 days of therapy as effective as 5 days? Please submit your answer in the form of a CAT; the main clinical bottom line should be derived from confidence interval data.

5. A 22-year-old, previously healthy college student is brought to the emergency room after sustaining a head injury in a campus touch football game. Witnesses state that he struck his head on the ground and was unconscious for "a few minutes." He has no known allergies and takes no medications. He denies headache, vomiting, or seizure after the injury. At the time he is seen in the emergency room, he is alert and oriented. His Glascow coma score is 15, and he is without focal neurological deficit on physical examination. Should a CAT scan of the head be performed?

6. You are asked to see a previously healthy 4-year-old child with a 2-week history of neck mass. The child was in her usual state of health until 2 weeks ago when she developed a low-grade fever and decreased appetite. At that time, her mother noted a small lump in the child's neck. Over the ensuing 2 weeks, the child has continued to have a low-grade fever, decreased appetite, and decreased activity. On physical examination, the vital signs are stable except for a temperature of 38°C. A 2 × 2 cm hard, nonmobile mass is noted in the lower anterior cervical region. Detailed examination of the lymphatics reveals bilateral anterior cervical as well as inguinal adenopathy. The liver is palpable 3 cm below the right costal margin.

INDEX